# Encyclopedia of Electromyography: Modeling and Analysis

## Volume III

# Encyclopedia of Electromyography: Modeling and Analysis
# Volume III

Edited by **Michael Backman**

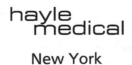

New York

Published by Hayle Medical,
30 West, 37th Street, Suite 612,
New York, NY 10018, USA
www.haylemedical.com

**Encyclopedia of Electromyography: Modeling and Analysis**
**Volume III**
Edited by Michael Backman

International Standard Book Number: 978-1-63241-161-7 (Hardback)

# Contents

# Preface

This book has been a concerted effort by a group of academicians, researchers and scientists, who have contributed their research works for the realization of the book. This book has materialized in the wake of emerging advancements and innovations in this field. Therefore, the need of the hour was to compile all the required researches and disseminate the knowledge to a broad spectrum of people comprising of students, researchers and specialists of the field.

Electromyography (EMG) is a technique for evaluating and recording the electrical activity produced by skeletal muscles. EMG is used for the diagnosis of neuromuscular issues and for determining biomechanical and motor control deficiency and other functional disorders. Moreover, it can be applied as a control signal for interfacing with orthotic and/or prosthetic devices or other rehabilitation aids. It will provide readers with a comprehensive introduction to EMG signal processing techniques and applications, while presenting several new results and explanation of existing algorithms. This book encompasses the analysis of theoretical and practical approaches of EMG research.

At the end of the preface, I would like to thank the authors for their brilliant chapters and the publisher for guiding us all-through the making of the book till its final stage. Also, I would like to thank my family for providing the support and encouragement throughout my academic career and research projects.

**Editor**

# EMG Modelling

# EMG Modeling

Javier Rodriguez-Falces, Javier Navallas and Armando Malanda

Additional information is available at the end of the chapter

## 1. Introduction

The aim of this chapter is to describe the approaches used for modelling electromyographic (EMG) signals as well as the principles of electrical conduction within the muscle. Sections are organized into a progressive, step-by-step EMG modeling of structures of increasing complexity. First, the basis of the electrical conduction that allows for the propagation of the EMG signals within the muscle is presented. Second, the models used for describing the electrical activity generated by a single fibre described. The third section is devoted to modeling the organization of the motor unit and the generation of motor unit potentials. Based on models of the architectural organization of motor units and their activation and firing mechanisms, the last section focuses on modeling the electrical activity of a complete muscle as recorded at the surface.

A mathematical model of a system describes the relations between a number of physical variables involved in the system. A mathematical model is a set of equations that can be implemented on a computer to study and to simulate the behaviour (response) of the system under specific conditions. EMG models presented in this chapter are structure based or structural, which means that they describe elements of the real biological structure and characterize them in a reductional way in order to represent the system's elements, behaviours or mechanism that are of importance. In the EMG models outlined here, the input variables or parameters are those that describe the anatomical, physiological, and functional properties of the biological structure under study (single fibre, motor unit, or entire muscle), whereas the output parameters are typically the extracellular generated potentials and/or specific quantitative measurements of these potentials.

Models of EMG activity are useful to address the "forward problem", that is, how specific mechanism and phenomena influence the generated potentials, as well as the "inverse problem", that is, how the extracellular potentials provide information about the underlying mechanism and phenomena. Accordingly, a desirable feature of an EMG model is that it allows studying the effect of the model's (input) parameters on the waveform of the potential, providing insight into the relationships between the anatomical and/or physiological properties of the fibre and the shape of the potential.

## 2. Modeling electrical conduction in skeletal muscle

Striated muscle is composed of a large number of striated muscle cells, also called muscle fibers. These elongated, cylindrical cells are arranged parallel to one another, and each one is surrounded by a plasma membrane called the sarcolemma. Muscle contraction is created via the repeated activation of several groups of muscle fibers, each of which is governed by a single motorneuron through its axon (Lieber, 2010). Figure 1(a) shows a portion of a muscle fiber that is attached, at the neuromuscular junction, to the terminal branch of its axon.

### 2.1. Depolarization and repolarization of a muscle fiber membrane

A muscle cell (fiber) is activated by electrical impulses coming from the motorneuron, which brings about the fiber's depolarization and the generation of a transmembrane voltage (normally defined as the extracellular electrical potential minus the intracellular one). Under normal conditions, the extracellular potential is practically zero, and so the transmembrane voltage can be considered to be practically the same as the intracellular action potential (IAP) (Burke, 1981; Plonsey and Barr, 2000). Membrane depolarization starts at the neuromuscular junction and extends along the muscle fiber towards both ends of the cell. As a result, two IAPs propagate without attenuation and with constant velocity $v$ along the muscle fiber towards the tendons, where they extinguish (Lieber, 2010).

The plasma membrane of a muscle fiber has the well-studied property of actively maintaining a nearly constant potential difference between the intracellular and extracellular environment. This voltage is normally referred to as the resting potential and has a value of about -80 mV [Fig. 1(b)]. The negative sign indicates that the interior is more negative than the exterior (negative polarization). In Fig. 1(a) the polarization of the fiber membrane is represented by a number of layers of negative signs. When the fiber is at rest, the number of negative layers remains unchanged. After fiber activation, two potential profiles (one at each side of the neuromuscular junction) arise along the fiber membrane. These profiles are normally referred to as waves of excitation, excitation sources or simply IAPs [Fig. 1(a)]. In Fig. 1(a) it can be seen that, along the spatial profile of the IAP, the number of negative-signed layers changes progressively with axial distance (the $x$-axis in Fig. 1). This reflects the fact that the IAP profile has gradual depolarization and repolarization transitions, as shown in Fig. 1(b).

### 2.2. The electric volume conduction

Knowledge of muscle fiber excitability and IAP propagation would be clinically useless if the electromyographist had to penetrate muscle fibers to obtain information about membrane processes. Moreover, recording of the IAP *in situ* from human muscle fibers has not yet proved feasible in EMG studies (Ludin, 1973). All electromyography (EMG) techniques are based on the fact that local electrophysiological processes result in a detectable flow of the transmembrane current at a certain distance from the active sources (i.e., muscle fibers). This flow of current in the tissue (i.e., the volume conduction), allows EMG measurements to be made at a distance from the sources.

The so-called *Principle of Volume Conduction* can be considered as a three-dimensional version of Ohm's law, which establishes that an electric current $I$, flowing between two points connected through a resistance $R$, generates a potential difference $V$ between these points: $V = I \cdot R$. In the case of living tissue, the electrical impedance is the inverse of the electrical conductivity $\sigma$. So, the potential recorded at a point $P_0$ ($x_0$, $y_0$, $z_0$) within an infinite volume with uniform conductivity $\sigma_i$ produced by a current $I_s$ injected in the same volume at a point $P$ ($x$, $y$, $z$) can be calculated as

$$V_{P_0} = \frac{1}{4\pi\sigma_i} \frac{I_s}{r_i} \tag{1}$$

where $r_i$ is the shortest distance between the points $P_0$ and $P$.

From inspection of (1), two main conclusions can be drawn. First, the potential recorded at a certain point is proportional to the strength of the current source, a feature highly desirable for electrodiagnostic medicine. Second, both $r_i$ and $\sigma_i$ are in the denominator of the equation (1). Thus, assuming a constant transmembrane current, the potential decreases with increasing radial distance and with increasing conductivity.

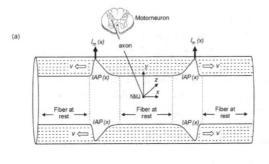

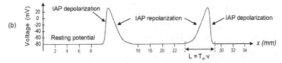

**Figure 1.** (a) Schematic representation of a portion of muscle fiber in which two excitation sources [IAP(x)] are propagating with velocity $v$ from the neuromuscular junction (NMJ) to the fiber ends. The polarization of the fiber membrane is represented by several layers of negative signs. The number of negative-signed layers within the fiber region delimited by the intracellular action potential (IAP) changes gradually with axial distance, but it is constant within the regions where the fiber is at rest. The transmembrane ionic electric current, $I_m(z)$, is also indicated. (b) Spatial profile of the IAP with its depolarization and repolarization phases. L and $T_{in}$ are the spatial extension and temporal duration of the IAP, respectively.

The principle of volume conduction is valid only as an intuitive approach to an understanding of the generation of an extracellular potential within a muscle. The simplicity of equation (1) hides important aspects that need to be clarified. First, the bioelectrical source cannot be described as a single injected current at a certain point, but it is rather a compound of multiple sources (see Section 3.1.2). Second, muscle fibers are of finite length, which implies that the assumption of an infinitely large volume conductor is never satisfied in practice. This will have important consequences: it will give rise to non-propagating components (see Section 2.2). Third, as muscle fibers can often be considered parallel to each other, conductivity of the muscle tissue in the longitudinal direction ($\sigma_x$) is higher than in the transversal ($\sigma_r$), i.e., the volume conductor is anisotropic with anisotropy ratio $K_{an} = \sigma_x/\sigma_r$.

## 3. Modeling the electrical activity of the single muscle fiber

In the last half of the 20th century EMG studies have directed attention to the calculation of single fiber action potentials (SFAPs) produced by excitable fibers and especially by fibers of finite length. The development of SFAP models was possible only after the principles of volume conductivity had been determined and the modelling of bioelectrical sources was well established.

### 3.1. Modeling the bioelectrical sources of muscle fibers

#### 3.1.1. The principles of bioelectricity

The principle of the electromotive surface proposed by Helmholtz in 1853 provided the basis for the electrical potential theory of volume conductors. In addition, he introduced the concept of an electrical double layer into the theory of electricity and suggested its use for the solution of certain boundary problems in electrical potential theory. The concept of the double layer (or dipole) source, however, went unused for about 30 years until Wilson et al. (1933) demonstrated its appropriateness for modelling the excitation source of a single circular cylindrical fiber. After Wilson, it was not until 1974 that Plonsey definitively clarified the underlying electrostatic principles of the single and double layer sources and related them to the concepts of monopole and dipole, respectively.

Traditionally, two kinds of sources (generators) have been considered in the literature (Lorente de No, 1947; Plonsey, 1974), namely, the "monopole" and the "dipole". A monopole is a single (point) source or sink of current within a conducting medium. It is quite rare that problems in bioelectricity involve monopoles, since all bioelectric generators involve at least source and sink combinations (Plonsey, 1974).

#### 3.1.2. A distributed presentation of the excitation source (excitation function)

Because of its propagation along the fiber, an IAP does not merely exist as a function of time: it also spreads out along the fiber as a function of space. The length of the IAP profile along the fiber, $L$, is defined by the product of the IAP duration, $T_{in}$, and the propagation velocity $v$ [Fig. 1(b)]. In fact, the formation of an electrical field around a fiber depends on the spatial extension of the IAP along the fiber (Dimitrova and Dimitrov, 2006; Rodriguez et al., 2011). In addition, the spatial profile of the IAP is smooth [Fig. 1(a)], implying that the electric properties of the fiber membrane affected by the IAP change gradually with axial distance. Accordingly, a correct presentation of the excitation function consists of a sequence of cylinders (fiber portions) of equally-infinitesimal length $dx$, each cylinder containing a density of sources, as represented in Figs. 2(b) and (c). If these sources are considered dipoles, then each of these cylinders should be represented by a double-layer disk [Fig. 2(b)], whereas if the sources are regarded as monopoles, then cylinders should be modeled as single-layer disks.

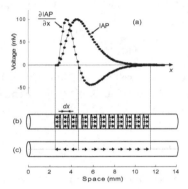

**Figure 2.** (a) Representation of the IAP spatial profile and its first spatial derivative, $\partial IAP/\partial x$. Schematic representations of the IAP as a sequence of double layer disks (b) (each disk comprising a density of dipoles), and as a sequence of lumped (point) dipoles (c) lying along the axis of the fiber.

From the above it follows that the calculation of the extracellular potential generated by a single excited fiber, $\Phi_e$, can be reduced to the sum of the potentials produced by a sequence of double (or single) layer disks distributed along the IAP spatial course (Dimitrova and Dimitrov, 2006). The specific mathematical derivation by which the extracellular potential is expressed in terms of double layer disks is presented below.

### 3.1.3. Calculation of the extracellular potential on the basis of dipoles

The dipole-based presentation of the source was first introduced by Wilson et al. (1933) and subsequently developed by Plonsey (1974). It is based on the hypothesis that the variation of the membrane electrical potential across an infinitesimal portion of the fiber membrane produces, in the extracellular medium, an electrical field that can be assumed to be equivalent to that produced by a lumped dipole (Wilson et al., 1933). So, the potentials produced by a double layer disk and a point dipole whose moment is proportional to the disk area are almost identical. This provides the basis for representing the portion of the fiber affected by the IAP as a sequence of dipoles distributed equidistantly along the IAP spatial profile (Dimitrova and Dimitrov, 2006; Rodriguez et al., 2011), as shown in Fig. 2(c). The strength of each of the dipoles (or dipole moment) is determined by the spatial derivative of the potential profile along the fiber $\partial IAP(x)/\partial x$. Orientation of the dipoles is determined by the sign of $\partial IAP(x)/\partial x$.

Let us consider a fiber element of infinitesimal length $dx$ of Fig. 2(b) lying within the region occupied by the action potential. A current emerges from this differential fiber element into the extracellular region. If we assume that all the current is concentrated along the fiber axis, then this current can be expressed as $\bar{p} \cdot dx$, where $\bar{p}$ is the dipole current per unit length. Since this current emerges essentially from a point into an unbounded space, it behaves like a point source of current (dipole generator) that lies in an extensive conducting medium. Then, the contribution to the extracellular potential generated from this component can be expressed as

$$d\Phi_e = \frac{1}{4\pi\sigma_e} \cdot \frac{d(1/r)}{dx} \cdot \bar{p}(x,t)dx \tag{2}$$

where $\sigma_e$ is the conductivity of the extracellular medium and $r$ is the distance from excitation source to the recording point, $P_0$ [see Fig. 3(e)]. If the element $\bar{p}\ dx$ is located at the coordinate $(x, y, z)$ and $P_0$ is located at $(x_0, y_0, z_0)$ then

$$r = \left[ (x-x_0)^2 + (y-y_0)^2 + (z-z_0)^2 \right]^{1/2} \tag{3}$$

Normally, the coordinate origin is placed on the fiber axis, whereupon $y = z = 0$. The total field produced in the extracellular medium by the propagation of a single dipole along the fiber is found simply by integrating with respect to x (i.e., summing up the contributions to the potential from the propagation of this single dipole current element). The result is

$$\Phi_e(x_0, y_0, z_0, t) = \int_{x=-\infty}^{x=\infty} \frac{\bar{p}(x,t)}{4\pi\sigma_e \cdot \left[ (x-x_0)^2 + y_0^2 + z_0^2 \right]^{3/2}} dx \tag{4}$$

At this point, we should remember that the source of excitation is actually a "distributed source", which means that we do not have just one dipole but a sequence of dipoles distributed equidistantly along the IAP profile. The distribution of the dipole moments (strengths) along the fiber axis is determined by the function $\partial IAP(x)/\partial x$. Thus, to be strictly correct, the actual source of excitation is a linear axial dipole source density

$$\bar{p} = -\pi a^2 \sigma_i \cdot \frac{\partial IAP}{\partial x} \cdot \bar{a}_x \tag{5}$$

where $\sigma_i$ is the intracellular conductivity and a is the fiber radius. If we now substitute (5) into (4), we obtain the dipole-based expression for the extracellular potential

$$\Phi_e(t) = -\frac{a^2 \cdot \sigma_i}{4 \cdot \sigma_e} \int_{-\infty}^{+\infty} \frac{\partial IAP(x,t)}{\partial x} \cdot \bar{a}_x \cdot \frac{\partial}{\partial x}\left(\frac{1}{r(x)}\right) dx \tag{6}$$

In (6) it can be seen that the term $\partial(1/r)/\partial x$ represents the scalar potential generated by a propagating dipole and the term $\partial IAP/\partial x$ corresponds to the distribution of moments of the collection of dipoles that form the excitation function.

Calculation of the extracellular potential on the basis of monopoles can also be derived following the steps outlined above, as shown in Plonsey and Barr (2000).

## 3.2. Models of the extracellular potential generated by a single muscle fiber

### 3.2.1. The first SFAP models

Lorente de Nó (1947) was the first to obtain an expression for the potential of the external field of a nerve in a volume conductor as a function of an action potential. However, he did not provide a physical interpretation for the concepts of double and single layer sources. Nevertheless, his contribution to the understanding and modelling of the extracellular fields produced by an excitable fiber in a volume conductor was essential for subsequent researchers.

In 1968, Clark and Plonsey proposed a SFAP approximation based on formal solutions of Poisson's or Laplace's equation with the corresponding boundary conditions using a method of separation of variables. The solution was based on the Fourier transform technique and modified Bessel functions. The formal solution, however, gave no opportunity for transparent physical interpretations (Andreassen and Rosenfalck, 1981). In addition, the mathematical expressions describing SFAPs using the volume conductor theory were quite complex, computationally time consuming and, therefore, somewhat unsuitable for simulating motor unit potentials (MUPs). In response to these limitations, simplified models were presented. The dipole and tripole models approximated the transmembrane current by two and three point sources, respectively. These models, however, presented important shortcomings. The dipole model was not able to describe the effects of the excitation origin and extinction correctly (George, 1970; Boyd et al., 1978; Griep et al., 1978). The tripole models failed to correctly describe SFAPs close to fibers (Griep et al., 1978; Andreassen and Rosenfalck, 1981).

### 3.2.2. Assumptions of the core-conductor model and the line-source model: the first approach to convolutional models

Clark and Plonsey (1966, 1968) and then Andreassen and Rosenfalck (1981), provided thorough compilations of the approaches that relate intracellular and extracellular potentials. Both works stressed the necessity of finding the conditions to simplify existing SFAP models. These conditions are summarized in the assumptions of the core-conductor:

a.   Axial symmetry is assumed. That is $\partial/\partial\phi=0$ (where $\phi$ is the azimuth angle) so that, at most, all field quantities are functions of the cylindrical coordinates only. In fact, transmembrane currents as well as intra- and extra-cellular potentials are considered to be functions only of $x$ (i.e., the core-conductor is linear).

b.  For a fiber in an extracellular medium of considerable extent, it is assumed that the resistance of the extracellular medium is practically 0, and so the influence of the medium surrounding the active fiber is neglected.

c.  The excitation source is assumed to be distributed along the axis of the fiber. Since in general fiber radius is many times smaller than fiber length, this approximation is normally justified.

On the basis of the volume conductor theory, Plonsey (1974) was the first to show that a SFAP can be expressed as a convolution of an excitation source and a weight function. An important step towards the simplification of this model was made by Andreassen and Rosenfalck (1981) who assumed that the transmembrane current was distributed and concentrated along the axis of the fiber (a line-source model). In addition, the authors theorized that the error caused by such a source simplification would be less than 5% provided the radial distance was 5 fiber radii or greater from the fiber axis. However, both the approach of Clark and Plonsey and that of Andreassen and Rosenfalck were still far from being simple and intuitive as they included an intricate mathematical formulation.

### 3.2.3. Towards an easy formulation of the SFAP convolutional model

After the key contributions of Clark and Plonsey and then Andreassen and Rosenfalck, great effort was directed towards including in SFAP models the effects of the finite size (Gootzen et al., 1991), inhomogeneneity (Dimitrova and Dimitrov, 2001), and frequency dependency (Albers et al., 1988) of the volume conductor. All of these authors were more interested in improving the accuracy of the SFAP model at the expense of reducing the physical transparency and the time efficiency of their approximations. However, these latter two considerations were precisely two features that scientists in other areas of EMG research and practice were increasingly demanding from SFAP models.

The key step towards an easy and intuitive presentation of the SFAP convolutional model was made by Nandedkar and Stalberg in 1983. The authors substituted the complex weight function used by Andreassen and Rosenfalck (that involved Bessel functions) for the simpler expression of a potential generated by a point current source (i.e., a monopole) that propagates along the fiber axis from the neuromuscular junction towards the tendons.

Although the Nandedkar and Stalberg model was found computationally more efficient and more accurate than the dipole and tripole models, it still lacked a suitable approach for dealing with the excitation onset and extinction. To overcome this problem, the excitation wave should be represented with two stacks of double-layer disks distributed equidistantly along the fiber axis. Following this idea, Dimitrov and Dimitrova (1998) replaced the stacks of distributed current dipoles by dipoles lumped along the axis of the fiber (line source model). The weight function was computed as the potential produced by two lumped current dipoles propagating in opposite directions from the endplate toward the fiber ends.

Let us assume that a unit dipole originates at time zero at the neuromuscular junction and propagates along a fiber with a constant velocity $v$. The potential produced by this unit dipole at the electrode is $IR(t)$ [Fig. 3(a)]. However, the source of excitation is actually a sequence of $n$

dipoles distributed equidistantly along the IAP profile, whose strengths (moments) are given by the function $\partial IAP(x,t)/\partial t$. The first dipole originates at time zero, and each subsequent dipole at an interval $\Delta t$. Let the amplitude of these dipoles be $a_1, a_2,..., a_n$ [Fig. 3(b)]. The first dipole originates at time zero, propagates towards the tendons, generating a potential $a_1 \cdot IR(t)$. The second dipole originates at time $\Delta t$, propagates towards the tendons, generating a potential $a_2 \cdot IR(t-\Delta t)$ [Fig. 3(c)]. Hence the total potential recorded by the electrode is

$$SFAP(t) = a_1 IR(t) + a_2 IR(t - \Delta t) + ... + a_n IR(t - (n-1)\Delta t) \qquad (7)$$

As $\Delta t$ tends to zero and $n$ tends to infinity, the total potential produced at the point $P_0$ by the propagating excitation function represents the convolution of $dIAP(x,t)/dt$ and $IR(t)$:

$$SFAP(t) = \frac{dIAP(t)}{dt} * IR(t) \qquad (8)$$

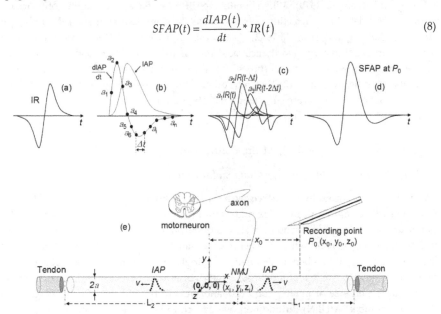

**Figure 3.** Presentation of the potential generated by a single fiber (SFAP) (d) as the output of a linear timeshift invariant system whose impulse response *IR* is the potential produced by a moving unit dipole (a) and whose input signal is a function of distributed dipoles whose strengths (moments) are determined by $dIAP(x,t)/dt$ (b). In (c) the contribution of each dipole to the total SFAP is shown separately. (e) Schematic representation of a muscle fiber innervated by the axon of a motorneuron.

Thus, an active fiber can be considered as a linear timeshift-invariant system for the generation of an extracellular potential. Specifically, the SFAP is the output of the system with the impulse response $IR(t)$ [Fig. 3(d)] and input signal $dIAP(x,t)/dt$. Since the activation of a skeletal muscle fiber gives rise to two oppositely-directed propagating IAPs, $IR(t)$ is the sum of potentials generated at the observation point by two dipoles moving in opposite directions from the neuromuscular junction to the fiber ends, where they disappear (McGill et al., 2001; Dimitrov and Dimitrova, 1998). This sum of potentials can be described as

$$SFAP(t) \;=\; K \cdot \int_0^t \frac{dIAP(\tau)}{d\tau} \cdot \frac{1}{v} \cdot \Big[ IR_1\big(t-\tau\big) + IR_2\big(t-\tau\big) \Big] \cdot d\tau \;=\; K \cdot \frac{1}{v} \cdot \frac{dIAP(t)}{dt} * IR\big(t\big) \qquad (9)$$

where * means convolution and $IR = IR_1 + IR_2$, $0 \le t \le t_{max}$. Constant $K$ is equal to $(a^2 \cdot \sigma_i)/(4 \cdot \sigma_e)$. The expressions for $IR_1$ and $IR_2$ and can be found in Dimitrov and Dimitrova (1998).

## 3.3. Models of electrodes for recording single-fibre potentials

The advent of single fiber electromyography (SFEMG) allowed investigators to analyze the shape peculiarities of the SFAP. The routine single fibre (SF) electrode consists of a montage of a 25-μm recording port (leading-off surface) referenced to the cannula (Ekstedt, 1964; Stålberg and Trontelj, 1979). When modelling SF electrodes, the leading-off surface is normally considered as a detection point, whereas the cannula is simulated through a plate electrode (Stalberg and Trontelj, 1992). As established by Ekstedt (1964), the conditions for recording an SFAP in a voluntarily activated muscle using an SF electrode are: (1) that the fibre is close to the electrode and thus gives rise to a potential with a short peak-to-peak interval (rise-time, RT), and (2) that any other fibres in the same motor unit that have coincident action potentials are sufficiently remote from the electrode that their contribution to the recorded signal is small.

## 4.1. Anatomy and physiology of the motor unit

### 4.1.1. Motoneuron, motor unit fibers, and motor unit territory

The motor unit is the entity that serves as a functional building block for the production of force and movement, both in reflex and voluntary contractions. Sherrington defined the motor unit as the set comprising a single motoneuron axon and the many muscle fibers to which that axon runs and which are hence innervated by it. The motor unit fibers (MUFs) are the different muscle fibers innervated by a single motoneuron. The numbers of muscle fibers supplied by a single motor neuron, through branching of its axons, is often referred to as the motor unit size or innervation ratio, and we will refer to this number as the motor unit fiber number (MUFN). In addition, we can consider the extent of the muscle cross-section that these fibers occupy, which is the motor unit territory (MUT), and the spatial distribution of these fibers within the motor unit territory area (MUTA). Subsequently, the motor unit can be characterization in terms of the motor unit fiber density (MUFD), measured as the number of MUFs per unit of area of its territory.

The MUFN varies greatly from one muscle to another and from one motor unit to another within the same muscle. The glycogen-depletion technique allows identification of the MUFs of a single motor unit within a muscle cross-section. Studies using this technique have demonstrated the large range of variation in MUFN (Burke and Tsairis, 1973), which extends from just a few fibers per motor unit in some muscles to thousands in others. Studies also show great variation within a single muscle: up to 100-fold from the smallest to the largest motor units.

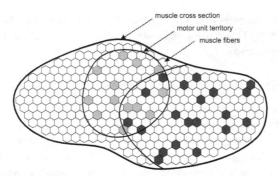

**Figure 4.** A schematic representation of the motor unit cross-section showing the MUFs of two motor units and delineating their MUTs which may overlap and may occupy only a fraction of the muscle cross-section.

By delineating the boundary enclosing the MUFs, we obtain a picture of the MUT. MUTs have been shown to be distributed over a localized region of a muscle's volume, with an approximately elliptical shape in cross-section [4] (see Fig. 4). That is, in terms of the muscle cross-section, only a fraction of its area is occupied by each motor unit (Bodine et al, 1988). This spatial feature was confirmed in humans using multilead-electrode-EMG, and using scanning-EMG (Stålberg and Antoni, 1980), with typical cross-sectional corridors between 5 and 10 mm long. Research based on glycogen-depletion techniques demonstrates that motor unit fibers of different motor units are intermingled, hence motor unit territories overlap within the muscle cross-section.

Defining the MUFD as the ratio of the MUFN to the MUTA, it is found that the ranges for MUFD are independent of the MUFN, while MUTA is strongly correlated with MUFN (Kanda and Hashizume, 1992). In reconstructions of the three-dimensional structure of motor units, MUFD is almost constant within a single motor unit when comparing the values obtained over the different cross-sections of the unit along the longitudinal axis of the muscle.

### 4.1.2. Spatial distribution of motor unit fibers

Another important feature related to motor unit fibers is their spatial distribution within the motor unit territory. Quantitative statistical studies in glycogen-depleted motor units by means of Monte Carlo simulation analysis (Bodine et al, 1988), suggest that MUFs are not homogeneously distributed: there are alternating regions of high and low MUF density within the MUT. High-density MUF areas are not usually located in the center of the MUT, as had been previously assumed. The various studies indicate that MUFs are arranged in small subclusters separated by holes with relatively few fibers, and researchers have suggested that if any clustering is present, it should be related to the axonal branching pattern established during development. The scanning EMG has confirmed the presence of silent areas within motor units of human muscles (Stålberg and Antoni, 1980), which most likely correspond to the holes observed in glycogen-depletion studies. Hence these results seem to agree with the long-range distribution findings in non-human vertebrates by the glycogen-depletion technique.

### 4.1.3. Motor end-plate zone, fiber diameter, and initiation of depolarization

Electrophysiologically, the motor end-plate is the region where the motor end-plate potential is generated, hence where the intracellular action potential of the muscle fiber starts. Thus, the relative longitudinal position of the motor end-plates of the set of muscle fibers belonging to a single motor unit is determinant in the synchronization of the single fiber action potentials. In addition, there will be different times for the initiation of the depolarization of the different motor end-plates, depending on the length of the axonal sprout innervating it. Besides, SFAPs will propagate at different conduction velocities through the muscle fiber, mainly dependent on muscle fiber diameter. All these factors (spatial configuration of end-plates, initiation of depolarization, and muscle fiber conduction velocity) affect synchronization of the SFAPs contributing to the MUP, and ultimately this will affect the shape, amplitude, and duration of recorded MUPs.

Neuromuscular junctions tend to reside in the middle part of muscle fibers, as the connection is established while a muscle fiber is still growing in both directions. The three-dimensional reconstruction of the motor end-plate zones leads to a two-dimensional membrane lying in the muscle volume. Measurements show that the width of this membrane, which corresponds to the variability in the longitudinal position of the individual motor end-plates, ranges between 6 and 10 mm in the *biceps brachii* (Aquilonious et al, 1984).

Muscle fiber conduction velocities can be measured *in situ* (Stålberg, 1966) and have a normal distribution of values for the whole of a given muscle. It is assumed that conduction velocity is directly proportional to fiber diameter, with histological analyses also showing a normal distribution for the diameters of muscle fibers.

Finally, a delay in the initiation of depolarization is caused by two factors: the axonal propagation delay, which is clearly dependent on the length of the axonal terminal branch and its propagation velocity; and the neuromuscular junction transmission delay, which has an average value, but also some variability (the "jitter").

## 4.2. Models for the motor unit cross section

The first computational muscle architecture models found in the literature were restricted to the simulation of a single motor unit. In essence, if individual motor units are modeled, of the triad: MUFN, MUTA, and MUFD, two quantities can be arbitrarily fixed, while the third will be a subsidiary quantity. After considering the dimensions and number of fibers of the motor unit, the models must deal with the placement of the individual MUFs within the MUT, in order to follow a certain spatial distribution.

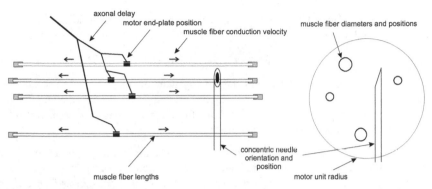

**Figure 5.** Representation of a simulated motor unit including the most relevant anatomical and physiological factor to reproduce the architecture and physiology of the motor unit.

The first motor unit model (Griep et al, 1978) was proposed in order to study the properties of the motor unit potential (MUP) by means of computer simulation. Other researchers, (Miller-Larsson, 1980; Gath and Stålberg, 1982; Hilton-Brown et al, 1985), were concerned with the modeling of fiber density and spatial distribution of muscle fibers of a single motor unit, in order to determine the influence of architectural changes produced by neuromuscular disease on clinical electrophysiological recordings. Other single motor unit models have been developed more recently. Other studies (Nandedkar et al, 1988; Stålberg and Karlsson, 2001) proposed a muscle model to study the correlation between anatomical parameters and MUP signals by means of simulations, allowing the study of the MUP variations under different pathological conditions such as denervation and re-innervation.

Two main approaches are used to model the spatial distribution of MUFs: random location and random selection from a muscle fiber grid. In the first approach, a number of MUFs are placed following a given spatial distribution, usually normal or uniform. In the second approach, a predefined grid of evenly distributed muscle fibers is created, and a number of them are selected to be innervated by the motor unit under simulation.

## 4.3. Models of the physiological parameters affecting the temporal dispersion of a MUAP

In all the above-mentioned models, muscle fiber conduction velocity, delay of initiation of depolarization, and longitudinal position of the motor end-plate are modeled as random variables from statistical distributions. It is important to note that, as individual motor units are being modeled, simulated distributions refer to the MUFs and not to all the fibers of the muscle bundle.

Muscle fiber diameter is modeled as a normally distributed variable with mean and standard deviation fixed to match corresponding values observed in real counterparts of the simulated muscle. Muscle fiber conduction velocity (MFCV) is modeled as a normally distributed variable, obtained from a linear transformation of the muscle fiber diameter. The most widely used relationship between fiber diameter and conduction velocity (Nandedkar and Stålberg, 1983) is:

$$v = 3.7 + 0.05 \, ( \, d - 55 \, ) \tag{10}$$

With v being the MFCV in m/s and d the muscle fiber diameter in μm. This equation assumes a linear relationship between both quantities, and a MFCV of 3.7 m/s for a muscle fiber diameter of 55 μm. Both these values are the central values of the corresponding distributions for the human *biceps brachii* muscle.

The delay in initiation of depolarization is usually modeled as a normal or uniform random variable, although in some cases its influence on simulation outcomes is assumed to be negligible and consequently it is not modeled and set to zero for all the muscle fibers.

Finally, the longitudinal position of the motor end-plates is modeled as a normal or uniform random variable, emulating the narrow width that the motor end-plate zone occupies within the longitudinal section of the muscle. Uniform distributions usually lead to overly complex MUPs, which seems to call for normal distributions. However, a specific model accounting for the motor unit fractions observed in scanning-EMG recordings, modeled the motor end-plates of small groups of motor unit fibers as narrower normal distributions with the mean of the distributions again distributed uniformly (Navallas and Stålberg, 2009). This model allows for a motor end-plate zone that is wider, whilst keeping the dispersion, and hence the MUP complexity, locally low.

## 4.4. Models of recording electrodes for intramuscular EMG

Point recording models, which are accurate enough for the simulation of single fiber EMG recordings, must be extended in order to simulate other needle electrodes where electrode poles are not small enough to be considered as points. Two main approaches are available. One is the analytical approach, which requires calculation of the integrals in order to simplify the calculations (Nandedkar and Stålberg, 1983; Dimitrov and Dimitrova, 1998). The other is the discrete elements approach, where the poles are modeled as grids of points where the potentials are calculated individually, and lately averaged to give the potential of the pole. In the case of concentric needle EMG, two poles must be modeled: the core, which represents the active recording region; and the cannula, used as the reference potential. The core, which is a small plane elliptical region, can be directly modeled using either approach. The cannula, a cylindrical region, which averages the potential over a much broader region than the core, can be simplified as a one dimensional cable structure coincident with the needle axis. In the case of macro EMG recordings, the active area is the cannula itself, and the electrode may be modeled accordingly.

There are other effects related to the needle insertion procedure that can also be modeled. Whenever the needle electrode is inserted, fibers in the way of insertion can be displaced by the needle shaft. This effect, named "fiber ploughing", calls for an update in the fiber positions according to the displacement suffered. The electrode manipulation typically performed by an electromyographist while recording concentric needle EMG can also be modeled. The electromyographist tries to bring the core closer to active fibers, producing sharp spikes in MUPs. In the corresponding model, the electrode is allowed to move 1 mm around the original insertion point in the longitudinal direction of the needle, and the position with the shortest distance to an active fiber is selected (Nandedkar et al, 1988; Hamilton-Wright and Stashuk, 2005).

## 5. Modeling electrical activity of skeletal muscle

In this section, the modeling of the electrical activity of a complete and functional muscle is described. After summarizing the principal anatomical and physiological characteristics of skeletal muscle, the different elements for building a model of a surface EMG signal generated by such a muscle are presented. Together with models of motor unit activity, discussed in the previous section, these elements comprise models for the architecture and geometric organization of the motor units within the muscle, models for the motor neuron pool activity, and models for the potentials recorded at the skin surface.

### 5.1. Physiological aspects concerning muscle EMG

In order to better understand the anatomical and physiological scenario which the models should recreate, an overview of the arrangement of MUs within the muscle and of the organization and strategies of the motor control is first provided.

*5.1.1. Anatomical and architectural organization of the motor units in skeletal muscle*

When trying to analyze a muscle's cross-section as a whole, overall statistics for the MUFN, MUTA and MUFD must be provided. We can think of the muscle cross-section as a tightly packed set of muscle fibers that are innervated by a smaller set of motoneurons. The innervation process, which determines the actual set of muscle fibers innervated by each motoneuron, defines the number and spatial distribution of the MUFs, hence the MUFN and the MUTA, and, subsequently, the MUFD.

The MUFNs of the motor units in a muscle tend to distribute exponentially, with fewer motor units with lower MUFN and less motor units with higher MUFN. Indirectly, MUFN can be studied on the basis of the mechanical response of the muscle. Studies of the mechanical response of skeletal muscle support the idea that many factors influence the force production of a single motor unit, including the MUFN, the cross-sectional area of motor unit fibers, and the specific tension output for the different muscle fiber types. However, within motor units of a single type, the main factor determining force production is shown to be the MUFN (Bodine et al, 1987). This makes it reasonable to assume that MUFN is proportional to motor unit maximum tetanic tension (Fuglevand et al, 1993). All these findings support the use of maximum tetanic force estimation techniques in order to investigate the MUFN in humans, where glycogen-depletion techniques obviously cannot be applied. The relative MUFNs can be assessed by measuring the sizes of the electrical and mechanical responses of individual motor units when motor axons are excited by threshold stimuli. Such a strategy involves determining the range of tetanic forces, and estimating the number of muscle fibers required to achieve these forces. These two parameters can be related by linear regression, which enables the estimation of MUFNs in human muscles.

Large ranges of variation of motor unit twitch force are found within single muscles, and the statistical distributions are shown to be highly skewed, with higher number of motor units with small motor unit twitch force, and lower number of motor units with large motor unit twitch force. Fuglevand et al. modeled the distribution of motor unit twitch forces by an exponential function (Fuglevand et al, 1993) that agrees highly with the experimental data (Kernell et al, 1983). Due to the high correlation found between MUFN and motor unit twitch tension, it can be assumed that an exponential function also governs the distribution of MUFN within motor units of a given pool.

The number of overlapping motor units at a given point of the muscle cross-section has been shown to range from 10 to 25 units in some human muscles (McIntosh, 2006). Glycogen-depletion studies have shown that the average MUTA differs for different motor unit types, in the order S<FR<FF, hence showing the same ordering as observed for MUFN. A strong positive correlation ($\varrho$ = 0.97) between MUTA and the maximum tension and a strong correlation between MUFN and motor unit maximum tension ($\varrho$ = 0.94) can be observed (Bodine et al, 1987). It is also found that the ranges for MUFD are different for each motor unit type and independent of the MUFN within each motor unit type, while MUTA is strongly correlated with MUFN within each motor unit (Kanda and Hashizume, 1992).

## 5.1.2. Hierarchical organization of motor control

Control of motor function is organized in three levels that act hierarchically and in parallel: the spinal cord, the brain stem and the motor areas of the cortex (Kandel, 1995). Each of these levels receives relevant sensory information from afferent pathways. This organization allows higher centres to give general commands, whilst leaving the control of detailed motor actions to lower level centres. The spinal cord is the lowest level of the hierarchy and contains neuronal circuits responsible for automatic motor patterns and reflexes. It contains a central region of grey matter that is occupied by millions of cell bodies of neurons of two types: interneurons and motor neurons (Guyton, 1994). Interneurons have many interconnections among themselves and with motor neurons, which form interneuronal circuits responsible for integration and feedback-based motor control functions. Motor neurons provide direct control of muscle activity by being directly innervated to muscle fibers. The MNs that innervate individual muscles are arranged in longitudinal columns forming what is known as the 'motor unit pool' (Kandel, 1995). The input to the motor neuron pool is the afferent information from peripheral receptors (muscle spindle, Golgi organs, Renshaw cells, etc.) and the efferent information (drive) from higher centres. The output of the motor unit pool consists on the firings of the different motoneurons in response to the different synaptic inputs they receive in the pool. Smooth coordinated movement relies on the subtle interplay of the command orders coming from the higher brain centers and the feedback information obtained by the peripheral receptors. Four interrelated mechanisms constitute the modulators of muscle activity: (1) MU recruitment, (2) motoneuron firing frequency (rate coding), (3) synchronization between pairs of MUs, and (4) the so-called 'common drive'. The first two are the principal gears of force modulation; while the other two are only secondary mechanisms for control of muscle force output.

## 5.1.3. Motor unit activation and firing strategies

### 5.1.3.1. Motor unit recruitment

Motor unit recruitment refers to the way in which the central nervous system selects the specific motor units to come into action as muscle force is required. Henemann and colleagues, in experiments on cats, observed an orderly recruitment of the motor neurons in the pool as the stimuli increased (Henneman, 1965). Specifically, smaller motor neurons were recruited before larger motor neurons. They refer to this behaviour as the 'size principle'. Many other works have reinforced the 'size principle', extending it to other species, different muscles and contraction tasks (Basmajian, 1985). Amplitude and conduction velocity of the MN impulses have been used as indirect indicators of motor neuron size. Twitch tension and MUAP amplitude have also shown strong positive correlation with recruitment order and spike amplitude (Merletti, 2004; Basmajian, 1985). As twitch tension and MUAP amplitude are known to be related to MU size, the 'size principle' indirectly links the order of the recruited MUs and their sizes.

The way recruitment is performed varies among muscles. In powerful muscles, such as the *biceps brachii* or deltoid, recruitment has been observed at least up to 80% maximal voluntary contraction (MVC) (Basmajian, 1985). On the other hand, in small muscles, as those of the hand, the pool of MUs is completely recruited for only 50% MVC. It has also been observed that when the voluntary force decreases, decruitment (deactivation of motor units) is performed in the opposite order to recruitment, in both isometric (De Luca, 1982) and dynamic contractions (Kossev, 1998).

### 5.1.3.2. Rate coding

Together with recruitment, rate coding is the most important mechanisms to modulate muscle force; the higher the discharge firing rate of a MU in a given task, the higher the force exerted by that MU. However different muscles and different contraction modalities exhibit different characteristics with respect to minimal and maximal firing frequencies and excitation-firing frequency curves (Basmajian, 85). Much of the current knowledge about recruitment and rate coding has been obtained thanks to the availability of reliable techniques for decomposition of MUAP trains from intramuscular EMG signals. One of these techniques is the so-called 'Precision Decomposition' technique, which was developed by De Luca and co-workers and included a recording system based on a quadrifilar needle electrode and programs to isolate several MUAP trains from the recorded signals (De Luca, 1993). With this system the researchers were able to track the evolution of several motor units in exercise protocols where force output was intended to follow a trajectory based on a linear increment, a constant level and a linear decrement. Various important paradigms of motor control could be formulated from the results of these experiments: (a) Lower threshold MUs tend to have lower initial firing rates than higher threshold MUs. (b) Earlier recruited MUs have higher firing rates than later recruited MUs. This occurs throughout the duration of the contraction, which gives rise to the typical 'onion skin' curves (Fig 6). (c) During sustained contractions the firing rates of MUs tend to decrease (De Luca 82) (Erim, 1996) (Fig 6). (d) The firing rate at decruitment is lower than at recruitment (Erim, 1996) (Fig. 6). (e) The firing rates of MUs with different thresholds tend to converge at maximum contractions (100% MVC).

All these findings indicate a hierarchy of MUs in the pool, which determines the recruitment order and the firing rates of MUs as a function of the required force (Erim, 1996).

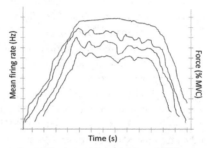

**Figure 6.** Schematic representation of the output force (red) and MUs mean firing rate evolution (Black) in an increasing ramp-sustained level decreasing ramp exercise.

Even in sustained contractions, the spikes of a MUAP train do not appear with an exact periodicity. The so-called interspike interval (ISI) variability is also an important aspect of rate coding (Merletti, 2004). When a MU is recruited, the ISI variability is relatively high and gets smaller as the firing rate increases (Basmajian, 1985).

### 5.1.3.3. Synchronization

MN synchronization refers to the "time-locked" spike trains delivered by two MNs in the pool over a certain time interval during a voluntary contraction. The "time-locked" (synchronous) pair of MUAP trains may be simultaneous or have a fixed lag, with a dispersion of a few milliseconds around the average lag (for example, of ±3ms (Sears, 1976) or ±5 ms (Datta, 1990). The number of synchronous spike pairs is more than what would be expected if the two MNs were discharging independently. Synchronization may have different neurological origins, but the most accepted one is the excitatory pre-synaptic potentials coming from brain stem descending neurons that branch into different motor neurons in the pool (Sears, 1976; Datta, 1990).

Using the cross-correlogram technique (Sears, 1976), Datta et. al. analyzed the synchronization of the first dorsal *interosseous* (FDI) muscle in isometric contractions and observed that the level of synchronization of two MU trains decreased as the difference between the recruitment thresholds of the two MUs increased (Datta, 1990). Kim *et. al.*

studied synchronization in four muscles under the conditions of slight isometric contraction and by means of two simultaneous intramuscular recordings (Kim, 2001). The selection of muscles for study was made in order to investigate proximal-distal and upper-lower dichotomies. Results showed synchronization in the four muscles, with higher degrees in distal relative to proximal muscles, and in muscles of the upper extremity relative to the lower. Analysis of synchronization in the frequency domain with the use of the coherence spectrum revealed coherence peaks in the 1-5 and 25-30 Hz bands, which indicated a common rhythmic input to the MN pool, probably related to oscillating activity in the brain and corticospinal projections (Kim, 2001).

*5.1.3.4. Common drive*

The tendency of the firing rates of different MU trains to fluctuate together in a low frequency range (1-2 Hz) over the course of contractions was first described by De Luca and his team (De Luca, 1982). They observed this common behaviour of MUs on FDI and deltoid muscles during sustained, linearly increasing and linearly decreasing contractions, and called it 'common drive'. They pointed to common excitatory inputs to several MUs in the pool as the probable origin of the phenomenon. Several subsequent studies evidenced similar effects in different muscles, with different exercises and in subjects of different ages (De Luca, 2002). Common drive has also been observed in muscles acting simultaneously in a certain task, either synergistically (De Luca, 2002) or in agonist-antagonist pairs (De Luca, 1987).

An interesting question is whether the phenomena of synchronization and common drive share a common origin. Semmler et al. recorded SEMG data from two separate fine-wire electrodes inserted into FDI muscles during slight isometric abduction. A low statistical correlation (<10%) between the indices that measured the extent of these processes was obtained (Semmler, 1997). Using simulated data, Jiang et. al. also studied the relationship between synchronization and common drive (Jiang, 2006). They found no correlation between the phenomena and a relationship of each of them to a different parameter in the proposed model (see Section 5.3.4, below). As Semmler et al., these authors concluded that synchronization and common drive must have a different physiological origin.

## 5.2. Models for muscle cross section

Several muscle architecture models have been proposed for EMG modeling. One of the objectives of these models is to reproduce the MUFN, MUTA, and MUFD distributions observed in real muscles. This implies modeling of the layout of the muscle fibers that form the muscle volume, sizing and placement of motor unit territories, and recreation of innervation patterns.

All models follow, to some degree, a common simulation scheme, depicted in Fig. 7. In order to compare the different models, we provide a classification of them based on the two components that most significantly affect the resulting properties of the models: the model of the motor unit territory placement, and the model of the innervation pattern. The different solutions proposed for each of the two components are identified. In addition, the parts which are common to most of the approaches are exposed.

The general procedure in all these models follows three main steps: (1) determination of the intended motor unit distributions (MUFN, MUFD, and MUTA); (2) placement of the MUTs; and (3) recreation of the innervation process by identifying the MUFs belonging to each of the motor units. In the following sections we will detail the different approaches available in these three steps.

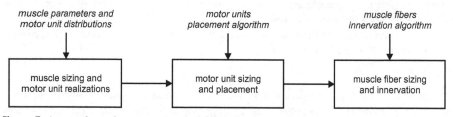

**Figure 7.** A general muscle cross-section model includes three steps in the simulation.

## 5.2.1. *Determination of the motor unit distributions*

Several parts of muscle architecture models tend to be common to all the available models. The geometry of the muscle is modeled by a cylinder with cross-sectional radius RMCS. Within the muscle cross-section, muscle fibers are assumed to be densely packed with a constant fiber density. Motor unit territories are modeled as circles on the muscle cross-section. Muscle fibers of different motor units are assumed to be intermingled, hence motor unit territories are allowed to overlap to a variable extent. To explain variation in maximum tetanic forces of motor units, physiological studies indicate a non-uniform distribution, which can be modeled by an exponential distribution (Fuglevand et al, 1993). If we accept that the number of muscle fibers within a motor unit is the main factor affecting the tetanic force variation (Bodine et al, 1997), we can assume, as well, an exponential distribution for the MUFN. A strong positive correlation between the MUFN and the MUTA has also been observed (Bodine et al, 1997). This seems to be consistent with a uniform value of the MUFD over the muscle cross-section. However, there is also evidence to suggest that MUFD distribution can depend on the motor unit type (Kanda and Hashizume, 1992). Hence, we should consider the assumption of constant MUFD as an approximation of the real properties of the entire motor unit pool. Accordingly, MUFD is usually assumed to be constant (20 fibers/mm$^2$, taking the value reported in (Burke et al, 1971)), and MUFN is assumed to follow an exponential curve:

$$n_i = \alpha \exp(\beta \, (i-1)) \quad ; i = 1, \ldots, N \tag{11}$$

where i is the motor unit index that ranks the motor units of a muscle from smaller to larger when sorted by the so called "size principle"; $n_i$ is the MUFN of the i-th motor unit; and $\alpha$ and $\beta$ are calculated to satisfy the MUFN range determined by $n_{min}$ and $n_{max}$ (the number of fibers in the smaller and larger motor units, respectively). The former equation is consistent both with the exponential distribution observed for the maximum tetanic forces of motor units, and with the linear relationship observed between the maximum titanic force and fiber number of motor units.

Finally, motor unit territory areas are usually calculated to fit both MUFN and MUFD, defined as MUFN/MUFD. In this way, as long as MUFD is assumed to be constant, MUTAs follow an exponential curve (Stashuk, 1993),

$$a_i = \alpha \, d_{MUF} \exp(\beta \, (i\text{-}1)) \quad ; i = 1, \ldots, N \tag{12}$$

where $a_i$ is the MUTA of the i-th motor unit, $d_{MUF}$ is the MUFD, and the rest of quantities are as given in (11). As MUTs are modeled as circles, (12) provides the means to calculate their radii.

### 5.2.2. MUT location: uniform, optimized, and developmental models

For motor unit territory placement, there are different approaches. The first three are based on independent uniform placement of territory centers within the muscle cross-section. Some authors (Fuglevand et al, 1993; Stashuk, 1993; Duchêne and Hogrel, 2000; Dimitrov et al, 2008) propose a uniform distribution of the territory centers within the muscle cross-section but with the restriction that the territories must lie completely inside the muscle cross-section. Other approach (Shenhav and Gath, 1986; Farina et al 2002; Keenan et al, 2006) is to consider a uniform distribution of the territory centers within the muscle cross-section, allowing the territories to partially exceed the muscle boundary and then cutting off the outlying part. A slight modification (Keenan and Valero-Cuevas, 2007) consists on assuming a uniform distribution of the territory centers within the muscle cross-section, allowing the territories to partially exceed the muscle boundary, cutting off the outlying part as in the previous model, and augmenting the territory radius until the inside region equals the original territory area. In general, these models tend to suffer from severe edge-effects, which lead to much higher MUT overlapping toward the center of the muscle cross-section than toward the edge (Navallas et al, 2009a; b). When the MUTs are cut-off, an additional effect of MUT area loss is present, leading to an increase of the MUFD beyond that intended (Navallas et al, 2009a; b). Although usually neglected, these effects severely affect the desired properties of the simulated muscle, and have to be taken into account.

Another approach, (Hamilton-Wright and Stashuk, 2005), is based on a seed-scattering algorithm. In this model, a grid of possible positions for the motor unit territory centers is created. The MUT center is placed at a seed position which is selected at random from this grid without replacement, and perturbed according to a bivariate normal distribution. When all the seed points have been used, the grid is replaced and the procedure of selecting the seed points without replacement begins again for the remaining MUTs. The resulting positions are refined during the innervation process such that they are the mean of the positions (center of mass) of the currently innervated muscle fibers. Similarly, the MUT radii are recalculated at the end of the innervation process.

The last approach considered here, (Schnetzer et al, 2001), consists in applying optimization algorithms to place the motor unit territories in such a disposition that the final muscle fiber density is as constant as possible. The authors presented two different algorithms. The first one places the motor unit territories at positions where the spatial variance of the muscle fiber density is minimized, and this algorithm can be used either with radius augmentation or without it. The second algorithm places the motor unit territories at positions where the muscle fiber density is minimal, and this approach can also be used with or without radius augmentation. These approaches ensure a uniform overlapping of the MUTs throughout the muscle cross-section, and a uniform muscle fiber density (Navallas et al, 2009b; 2010), which are desired properties for any muscle architecture model. As with the uniform models, cutting-off the MUTs leads to a loss of MUT area with negative effects on the simulation of the MUFD (Navallas et al, 2009b). Therefore, cut-off should be avoided in favor of the "augmented radius" versions of the algorithms.

### 5.2.3. MUF innervation: scatter, random, and weighted models

In the literature, some models explicitly state the algorithm used to model the innervation process. In these models, prior to innervation, a square or hexagonal grid of muscle fibers is created within the muscle cross-section. Then, for each of the muscle fibers, an innervating motor unit is selected from the set of units whose territories cover the fiber position. This assignment can be done in a completely random manner (Stashuk, 1993) or by weighting the innervation probabilities. The idea behind such assignments is to model non-homogeneous distributions of muscle fibers within the motor unit territory (Cohen et al, 1987; Hamilton-Wright and Stashuk, 2005; Navallas, 2010), or to control the number of innervated fibers (Hamilton-Wright and Stashuk, 2005). A further refineed algorithm (Navallas, 2010) uses an analytical expression of the probability distributions of the outcomes (MUFN, MUFD, and MUTA) to determine the innervation probabilities in order to satisfy certain target distributions.

Other approaches simply state that muscle fibers of a given motor unit are scattered within the motor unit territory (Duchêne and Hogrel, 2000; Stålberg and Karlsson, 2001; Farina et al, 2002; Dimitrov et al, 2008; Keenan et al 2006) with no prior grid of muscle fibers within the muscle cross-section. Often, papers describing scatter models do not provide the algorithms used for the placement of the motor unit fibers within the motor unit territory. The reader might guess that one of two possible approaches have been used: we can assume that the exact number of motor unit fibers is assigned to each motor unit, or that the number of motor unit fibers assigned to each motor unit is calculated to satisfy the expected MUFD. Note that, as long as MUTA remains unchanged, both approaches would be equivalent. In both cases, the final motor unit fiber positions can be obtained at random from a uniform distribution over the motor unit territory. This approach should imply the use of a particular mechanism to avoid collisions between muscle fibers, solving the so called "fiber packing problem".

All of these models are adequate as long as optimized-augmented MUT placement has been carried out previously (Navallas et al, 2009b). However, only the inverse-model for weighted innervation ensures that exactly the intended MUFN, MUFD, and MUTA distributions will be obtained for the simulated muscle (Navallas et al, 2010).

### 5.2.4. Motor unit temporal dispersion parameters

If whole-muscle distribution characteristics are used in modeling the distributions of muscle fiber conduction velocities and motor end-plate locations of the motor unit, the result is usually overly complex MUPs. Muscle fiber diameters can be modeled to follow a normal distribution within individual motor units but with an increasing mean and standard deviation as a function of the motor unit index (Hamilton-Wright and Stashuk, 2005). The rationale behind this approach lies in the differences in diameters of fibers of different types. With this approach, the variability in muscle fiber conduction velocities within individual motor units is narrower, leading to more accurate levels of MUP complexity, while the overall distribution for the whole muscle follows a wider and almost normal distribution, as expected.

Generally, the approach to modeling end-plate locations is the same as that used for individual motor units, hence drawing the locations from normal or uniform distributions as described in section 3.3. Thus, end-plate locations are assumed to be uncorrelated between different motor units. However, more complex approaches (Navallas and Stålberg, 2009) can also be used to ensure further realism in the degree of complexity of the simulated MUPs, although end-plate locations are always independent from one motor unit to another.

Axonal delays and the mean neuromuscular transmission delay, as in the case of single motor units, are usually neglected and left unmodeled. However, in more accurate models (Hamilton-Wright and Stashuk, 2005), the neuromuscular junction transmission delay variability is accommodated. This model of "jitter" values, in which individual transmission delay variability can be modeled using the actual values found in real single-fiber EMG recordings, provides simulated jitter values that are highly correlated with those observed in reality.

## 5.3. Modeling motor unit activation and firing strategies

### 5.3.1. Models for recruitment

Given a set of motor units of known sizes in the pool, the 'size principle' straightforwardly defines the order in which these motor units will be recruited with increasing excitation and decruited with decreasing excitation. The model, explained in (Fuglevand, 1993) and applied in other simulation studies (Yao, 2000; Farina, 2002; Zhou 2004; Gabriel 2009), aims to configure the recruitment threshold excitation (RTE) so that many MUs are assigned low thresholds, while relatively few MUs are assigned high thresholds. An exponential law similar to equation (XX) for the distribution of MUFN in the pool (see Section 5.2.1), was proposed for the RTE values. A motoneuron will remain inactive as long as the excitation target force (Fuglevand, 1993) or torque (Farina, 2002) level in the pool is lower than the motoneuron's threshold, and will start firing when the excitation level reaches that threshold.

A new perspective for recruitment modelling was offered by Wakeling (2009), who introduced two input functions, one excitatory and one inhibitory, for governing recruitment. When the excitation (demanded force) is increased from zero to a maximum level, this mechanism produces the recruitment of motor units of increasingly higher thresholds and the decruitment of motor units with low thresholds.

## 5.3.2. Models for rate coding

Rate coding models are characterized by three different elements concerning the pool of MUs: the minimum firing rate, the excitation-firing rate curves and the inter-spike interval (ISI) variability (Fuglevand, 1993).

### Minimum. firing rate

Although there is a tendency for lower threshold MUs to have lower initial firing rates than higher threshold MUs (Erim, 1996), minimum firing rates are similar for all MUs in the pool (Monster, 1977; Fuglevand, 1993). In (Fuglevand, 1993; Yao 2000; Farina 2002; Zhou 2004) the minimum firing rate was given a constant value of 8 Hz for the whole pool of MUs.

### Excitation-firing. rate curves

After the experimental work of Milner Brown (1973), the relationship between the firing rate of the MUs of the pool and the excitation has been modelled by means of a linear function (Fuglevand, 1993; Yao 2000; Farina 2002; Zhou 2004). Different behaviours in relation to the peak firing rates (PFR) of MUs, in combination with the slope of the excitation-firing rate curves (SEFRC), has led to different models for these curves:

a.  SEFRC is the same for all MUs, and PFRs are in inverse proportion to the recruitment threshold (Fuglevand, 1993; Zhou, 2004) (Fig 8.A). This model is based on observations made in cats, monkeys and humans (Fuglevand, 1993) and is consistent with the 'onion skin' phenomenon (Erim, 1996).
b.  SEFRC is the same for all MUs and the PFR is the same for all the MNs in the pool (Fuglevand, 1993; Farina 2002) (Fig 8.B). Several experimental works support this strategy (Fuglevand, 1993).
c.  SEFRC is the same for all MUs and PFRs are proportional to MU recruitment thresholds (Fuglevand, 1993; Zhou, 2004) (Fig 8.C). In this case, peak firing rates are related to the mechanical outputs of the MUs in the sense that large force, fast contracting MUs are assigned higher PFRs than small force, slow contracting MUs. This model is also based on experimental observations (Fuglevand, 1993).
d.  SEFRC increases with the recruitment threshold, so that all MUs finally reach the same PFR at maximum excitation (Zhou, 2004) (Fig 8.D).

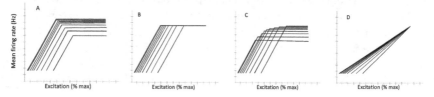

**Figure 8.** Linear excitation-firing rate curves.

### ISI. variability

In most cases a Gaussian distribution has been confirmed to best fit the experimental data (Merletti, 2004; Fugglevand, 1993). But, a Poisson distribution and a gamma distribution have also been proposed (Merletti, 2004).

*Physiological. models for the MU firing rate*

A different model for firing rates of MUs was proposed by Matthews (1996). He considered that the repolarization phase of the membrane potential could be modelled by an exponential curve. When this curve crosses a certain threshold, a new action potential is fired. This leads to the repetitive firing of action potentials with a constant firing rate, which depends on the exponential decaying factor and on the threshold. Higher thresholds would lead to higher firing frequencies and *vice versa*. White Gaussian noise of zero mean was superimposed on the membrane exponential curves, thus introducing variability into the interspike intervals, which was directly related to the power of the noise.

Jiang et al. (2006) proposed a model for the generation of action potential trains in a small set of neurons, which included excitation neurons, motoneurons and synapses. In the particular example developed, one excitation neuron provided common input signals to two different MUs through corresponding synapses, which also received feedback information from the MN outputs (Fig 9). To compare the outputs of the model to data from real experiments, SEMG recordings were obtained from *biceps brachii* and *abductor pollicis brevis* muscles during slight isometric contractions. Real and simulated signals showed similar results regarding MN synchronization and common drive (see below).

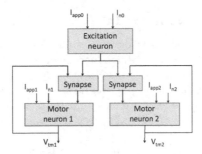

**Figure 9.** Jiang's model for the generation of action potential trains. $I_{app}$: applied currents, responsible of the neuron excitability, $I_n$: noise currents, $V_{tm}$: output potentials.

## 5.3.3. Models for synchronization

Yao et. al. proposed a model for MU synchronization which basically adjusts the firing instants of MUs in the pool so that they attain a certain degree of time proximity among them (synchronization) (Yao, 2000). This model is used to study the influence of synchronization on SEMG and output force as the neural excitations varies. Simulation results show that both the SEMG level and the variability of output force increase with synchronization, but the level of output force itself is not significantly influenced by it. The same conclusions were reported in the simulation study carried out by Zhou et. al. (2004)using Yao's model. This model was also used by Gabriel and Kamen (2009) in their inverse modelling study conducted to find out the physiological strategies responsible for elevating the force level in isometric voluntary contractions in *biceps brachii*. They concluded that either rate coding or synchronization could provide output data fit to the real data and that either of these two strategies, or a combination of the two, could be involved in the motor process.

A different model was proposed by Kleine et al. (2001), who slightly modified Matthews' firing rate model to introduce synchronization in a controlled way. In essence, the noisy input component is divided into two parts, one which is common to other MUs in the pool and one that is unique and independent of the other MUs. Simulation of SEMG signals correctly predicted the findings observed experimentally in isometric contractions of the trapezius muscle.

### 5.3.4. Modeling the common drive

Jiangs' physiological model for modeling the generation of MN firing trains also enables the simulation of common drive (Jiang, 2006). In the example explored (Fig. 9), there are independent MN inputs that determine their excitabilities ($I_{app1}$ and $I_{app2}$). When these inputs are given a common oscillating signal, emulating interneural or afferent signals reaching the two MNs, their firing rates exhibit a clear correlation (common drive), although synchronization is not appreciably affected.

## 5.4. Models for the potentials recorded at the skin surface

Models for the potentials recorded at the skin surface usually follow the convolutional approach, that is, they try to find a 'weighting function' that provides the potential recorded at any point on the surface of the skin above the active fiber and caused by an elementary current source at the fiber. First of all, a geometric model of the muscle has to be defined, which might accommodate the existence of several tissue layers with different electrical properties (conductivities and capacitances). Together with the 'weighting function', a source function of the distribution of current sources in the fiber, such as one of those proposed for the single fiber case (Rodríguez et al, 2012), has to be used. Apart from the infinite homogeneous volume conductors, one of the first approximations for modeling the geometry of the muscle was the semi-infinite structure, which divides the complete (infinite) space into two parts separated by the skin plane: one with finite conductivity representing the muscle tissue, and one with zero conductivity, representing the other side of the skin plane (Merletti et al, 1999).

Muscle tissue presents higher conductivity in the direction longitudinal to the fibers than in the perpendicular direction. To include this behaviour into EMG models a new coefficient was included in the formulation of the 'weighting function': the anisotropy ratio (ratio between conductivities in the longitudinal and perpendicular directions) (Merletti et al, 1999). The effects of fat and skin layers, that have different electrical properties (conductivity and capacity), have also been incorporated into some models (Farina, 2001), (Block, 2002; Lowery 2002). The fat layer is normally considered isotropic, with conductivity appreciably lower than the muscle. Skin has a laminar structure with a highly resistant stratum corneoum and a deeper granular tissue with higher conductivity. However, it is normally modelled as a simple layer with homogeneous conductivity, although there is not general agreement about the values of skin conductivity ), (Block, 2002; Lowery 2002). The effects of these layers have been studied through simulation; relative to models which only include one or two layers, multi-layer models generate potentials with peak amplitudes closer to those found in real recordings.

An important step forward in the construction of more elaborated EMG models is the inclusion of finite limb geometries. Cylindrical muscle models have been developed by several authors (Gootzen, 1989; Roeleveld, 1997; Farina, 2004) in which the fibers run parallel to the cylinder axis. But, fibers may also run radially within a cylindrical geometry, for example, in the anal sphincter (Farina, 2004) or have different fiber-pinnation angles (Mesin, 2004). More complicated geometries, which include bones and vessels, have also been included in the models (Mesin, 2008). As the geometrical structure and composition of layers of the EMG model is made more complicated, defining and solving the electrical equations of the problem becomes more difficult. Iterative computational approaches such as the finite-element method (FEM) or boundary element method (BEM) are called for. In (Lowery, 2002) a FEM model with cylindrical geometry was devised for a muscle. This included the muscle tissue, fat and skin layers and a bone, all of them with specific conductivities. Similarly, a FEM model with a realistic geometry taken from magnetic resonance images of a particular subject's muscle was also modelled (Lowery, 2004). Simulated signals from both models were compared to real EMG data from electrical stimulation of the upper arm. Both models presented similar features with regard to peak amplitude and power spectrum mean frequency as functions of the recording position. However, the more realistic model (Lowery, 2004) provided action potential shapes closer to those actually recorded (Lowery, 2002).

Finally, the effects of the surface EMG electrodes potentials should also be included in the model. In general, placing an electrode on the skin surface does not alter the potential field. This is due to the relatively high impedance "seen" by the conductor tissue, which is, in turn, due to the electrochemical double layer formed between the metal of the electrode and the tissue. The potential recorded by the electrode is then the average potential in the surface covered by the electrode (McGill, 2004). Analytical or numerical procedures may be used to calculate this average either in the spatial domain (Dimitrov, 1998; Merletti, 1999) or in the spatial frequency domain (Farina, 2004).

## 5.5. Conclusions and open research lines

A general perspective of EMG modeling has been displayed together with a description of the anatomical and functional physiological aspects, in which the described models are grounded. This panoramic view comprises models for the space and size distribution and architectural organization of MUs in the muscle; a view of the hierarchical organization of the motor control; models for the principal MU activation and firing strategies for muscle force production: MU recruitment, 'rate coding', MN synchronization and the 'common drive'; and models for the generation of potentials at electrodes placed on the skin surface.

Experimental research works sustaining evidences for the theories and concepts described in the chapter have also been included.

The research effort in modeling and simulating EMG signals in the last three decades has been paramount including both analytical as well as numerical orientations. The degree of complexity and detail has also run parallel to these developments with the aim of recreating the physiological EMG generation system on one hand and the temporal and spectral features of real EMG signals on the other hand. However, there is still room for improvement in several aspects:

-   Most experimental observations related to force modulation mechanisms are referred to isometric contractions. The extent of the validity of existing models of such mechanisms in dynamic contractions is not solidly established yet, deserving more research attention.
-   SMEG generation models with increasingly complex muscle geometry and fibers disposition have been developed (Messin 2004; Messin 2008; Lowery 2002). On the other hand, sophisticated models for the MU geometrical distribution and MUF innervations have been put forward (Navallas 2010). However, these two different and complementary modeling pieces have not been put together yet, as a unified approach of muscle architecture. Their combination could represent even better the complex physiological arrangement of fibers and MU in the muscle, permitting more refined simulation studies.
-   The phenomena of MU substitution (Westgaard, 1999) and replacement (Bawa, 2009), which appears in prolonged contractions, can be considered as a fifth strategy for MU firing rate control. EMG models that include these phenomena are still missing.
-   Fatigue, aging and neuromuscular disease are specific circumstances that degrade muscle performance. EMG models for these situations are scarce (Dimitrov, 2008; Nandedkar, 1989; Stalberg 2001; Enoka, 2003) but may be indeed very useful for better understanding the underlying mechanisms. More research attention should therefore be given to this important area of EMG modeling.

## Author details

Javier Rodriguez-Falces, Javier Navallas and Armando Malanda
*Department of Electrical and Electronic Engineering, Public University of Navarra, Pamplona, Spain*

## 6. References

Albers, BA., Rutten, WLC., Wallinga, W., & Boom, HBK. (1988). Frequency domain modelling of volume conduction of single muscle fiber action potentials. *IEEE Trans Biomed Eng*, Vol. 35, pp. 328-333.

Andreassen, S., & Rosenfalck, A. (1981). Relationship of intracellular and extracellular action potentials of skeletal muscle fibers. *CRC Crit Rev Bioeng*, Vol. 7, pp. 267–306.

Aquilonius, SM., Askmark, H., Gillberg, PG., Nandedkar, S., Olsson, Y. & Stålberg, E. (1984) Topographical localization of end-plates in cryosections of whole human muscles. *Muscle Nerve*, Vol. 7, pp. 293–297.

Arai, T. & Kragic, D. (1999). Variability of Wind and Wind Power, In: *Wind Power*, S.M. Muyeen, (Ed.), 289-321, Scyio, ISBN 978-953-7619-81-7, Vukovar, Croatia

Basmajian, JV. & De Luca JC. (1985). Muscles alive. Their function revealed by Electromyography. Baltimore, USA: Williams and Wilkinson.

Bawa, P., Murnagham, C. (2009). Motor unit rotation in a variety of human muscles. J Neurophysiology 102, pp. 2265-2272.

Block, J.H., Stegeman, D.F. & Van Oosterom, A. (2002) Three-layer volume conductor model and software package for applications in surface Electromyography. *Annals Biomed Eng.* Vol. 30. pp. 566-577.

Bodine, SC., Garfinkel, A., Roy, RR. & Edgerton, VR. (1988) Spatial distribution of motor unit fibers in the cat soleus and tibialis anterior muscles: local interactions. *J Neurosci*, Vol. 8, pp. 2142-2152.

Bodine, SC., Roy, RR., Eldred, E. & Edgerton, VR. (1987) Maximal force as a function of anatomical features of motor units in the cat tibialis anterior. *J Neurophysiol*, Vol. 57, pp. 1730-1745.

Boyd, DC., Lawrence, PD., & Bratty, PJA. (1978). On modeling the single motor unit action potential. *IEEE Trans Biomed Eng*, Vol. 25, pp. 236–43.

Burke, RE. & Tsairis, P. (1973) Anatomy and innervation ratios in motor units of cat gastrocnemius. *J Physiol*, Vol. 234, pp. 749-765.

Burke, RE. (1981). Motor units: anatomy, physiology and functional organization. In: *Handbook of Physiology. The Nervous System. Motor Control*, pp. 345–422, Bethesda, MD: American Physiological Society.

Burke, RE., Levine, DN. & Zajac, FE. (1971) Mammalian motor units: physiological-histochemical correlation in three types in cat gastrocnemius. *Science*, Vol. 174, pp. 709-712.

Clark, J., & Plonsey, R. (1966). A Mathematical Evaluation of the Core ConductorModel. *Biophys J*, Vol. 6, No 1, pp. 95–112.

Clark, J., & Plonsey, R. (1968). The Extracellular Potential Field of the Single Active Nerve Fiber in a Volume Conductor. *Biophys J*, Vol. 8, No. 7, pp. 842–864.

Cohen, MH., Lester, JM., Bradley, WG., Brenner, JF., Hirsch, RP., Silber, DI. & Ziegelmiller, D. (1987) A computer model of denervation-reinnervation in skeletal muscle. *Muscle Nerve*, Vol. 10, pp. 826-836.

Datta, AK., Stephens, JA. (1990). Synchornization of motor unit activity during voluntary contractions in man. *J. Physiol. Lond.* Vol. 442, pp 397-419.

De Luca JC. (1993). Precision decomposition of EMG signals. *Meth Clin Nueurophysiol*. Vol 4. pp. 1-28.

De Luca, JC. & Erim, Z. (2002). Common drive in motor units of a synergistic muscle pair. *J. Neurophysiol*. Vol. 87, pp 2200-2204.

De Luca, JC. & Mambrito, B. (1987). Voluntary control of motor units in human antagonist muscles: coactivation and reciprocal activation. . *J. Neurophysiol*. Vol. 58, pp 525-542.

De Luca, JC., LeFever, RS., McCue, MP & Xenakis, P. (1982). Controls scheme governing concurrently active hunan motor units during voluntary contractions. *J. Physiol.* Vol. 329, pp 129-142.

Dimitrov, GV., & Dimitrova, NA. (1998). Precise and fast calculation of the motor unit potentials detected by a point and rectangular plate electrode. *Med Eng Phys,* Vol. 20, pp. 374–381.

Dimitrov, GV., Arabadzhiev, TY., Hogrel, JY. & Dimitrova NA. (2008). Simulation analysis of interference EMG during fatiguing voluntary contractions. part I: What do the intramuscular spike amplitude-frequency histograms reflect? *J Electromyogr Kinesiol,* Vol. 18, pp. 35-43.

Dimitrova, NA., & Dimitrov, GV. (2006). Electromyography (EMG) modeling. In: *Wiley encyclopedia of biomedical engineering.* Metin A, Hoboken, NJ: John Wiley & Sons.

Dimitrova, NA., Dimitrov, AG., & Dimitrov, GV. (1999). Calculation of extracellular potentials produced by inclined muscle fibers at a rectangular plate electrode. *Med Eng Phys,* Vol. 21, pp. 582–587.

Dimitrova, NA., Dimitrov, GV., & Dimitrov, AG. (2001). Calculation of spatially filtered signals produced by a motor unit comprising motor unit with a non-uniform propagation. *Med Biol Eng Compt.* Vol. 39, pp. 202–207.

Duchêne, J. & Hogrel JY. (2000) A model of EMG generation. *IEEE Trans Biomed Eng,* Vol. 47, pp.192-201.

Ekstedt, J. (1964). Human single fibre action potentals. *Acta Physiol Scand,* Vol. 61, No. 226, pp. 1-96.

Enoka RM, Christou EA, Hunter SK, Kornatz KW, Semmler JG, Taylor AM, Tracy BL. (2003) Mechanisms that contribute to differences in motor performance between young and old adults. J Electromyogr Kinesiol. Feb;13(1):1-12.

Erim, Z., De Luca CJ., Mineo, K. & Aoki, T. (1996). Rank-ordered regulation of motor units. *Muscle & Nerve.* Vol. 19. pp. 563-573.

Farina, D., Cescon, C. & Merletti, R. (2002) Influence of anatomical, physical, and detection-system parameters on surface EMG. *Biol Cybern,* Vol. 86, pp. 445-456.

Farina, D., Fosci, M. & Merletti, R. (2002). Motor unit recruitment strategies investigated by surface EMG variables. *J. Appl Physiol.* Vol. 92, pp 235-247.

Farina, D., Mertetti, R. (2002). A novel approach for precise simulation of the EMG signal detected by surface electrodes. *IEEE Trans Biomed Eng,* Vol. 48, pp. 637-646.

Farina, D., Messin, L., Martina, S., Mertetti, R. (2004). A surface EMG generation model with multilayer cylindrical description of the volume conductor. *IEEE Trans Biomed Eng,* Vol. 51, pp. 415-426.

Fuglevand, AJ., Winter, DA. & Patla, AE. (1993) Models of recruitment and rate coding organization in motor-unit pools. *J Neurophysiol,* Vol. 70, pp. 2470-2488.

Fuglevand, AJ., Winter, DA., Patla, AE., & Stashuk, D. (1992). Detection of motor unit action potentials with surface electrodes: influence of electrode size and spacing. *Biol Cybern,* Vol. 67, pp. 143–53.

Gabriel, DA., Kamen, G. (2009). Experimental and modelling investigation of spectral compression of biceps brachii SEMG activity with increasing force levels. *J Electromyogr Kinesiol.* Vol. 19. pp. 437-448.

Gath I. & Stålberg E. (1982) On the measurement of fibre density in human muscles. *Electroencephalogr Clin Neurophysiol,* Vol. 54, pp. 699-706.

George, RE. (1970). The summation of muscle fiber action potentials. *Med Biol Eng,* Vol. 8, pp. 357–65.

Gootzen, T., Stegeman, D., & Van Oosterom, A. (1991). Finit limb dimensions and finite muscle length in a model for the generation of electromyographic signals. *Electroenceph Clin Neurophysiol,* Vol. 81, pp. 152-162.

Gootzen, TH., Stegeman, DF. & Heringa A. (1989). On numerical problems of analytical calculation of extracellular fields in bounded cylindrical volume conductors. *J. Appl Physiol.* Vol. 66, pp. 4504-4508.

Griep, PAM., Boon, KL. & Stegeman, DF. (1978) A study of the motor unit action potential by means of computer simulation. *Biol Cybern,* Vol. 30, pp. 221-230.

Guyton AC. (1994). Anatomía y fisiología del sistema nervioso (2ª edición). Madrid, España. Editorial Médica Panamericana.

Hamilton-Wright, A. & Stashuk, DW. (2005) Physiologically based simulation of clinical EMG signals. *IEEE Trans Biomed Eng,* Vol. 52, pp. 171-183.

Helmholtz, H. (1853). Messungen über einige Gesetze der Vertheilung elektrischer Ströme in Körperlichen Leitern mit Anwendung auf die thierischelektrischen Versuche Ann Physik u Chem, Vol. 89, pp. 211–353.

Henneman, E., G. Somjem & D. O. Carpenter. (1965). Functional significance in cell size in spinal motoneuros. *J. Neurophysiol.* Vol. 28, pp 560-580.

Hilton-Brown, P., Nandedkar SD. & Stålberg EV. (1985) Simulation of fibre density in single-fibre electromyography and its relationship to macro-EMG. *Med Biol Eng Comput,* Vol. 23, pp. 541-546.

Hodgkin, AL., & Huxley, AF. (1952). A quantitative description of membrane current and its application to conduction and excitation in nerve. *J Physiol,* Vol. 117, pp. 500-544.

http://sciyo.com/articles/show/title/wind-power-integrating-wind-turbine-generators-wtg-s-with-energy-storage

Jiang, N., Parker, PA., Englehart, KB. Modeling of muscle motor unit innervation process correlation and common drive. *IEEE Trans Biomed Eng,* Vol. 53, pp. 1605-1614.

Kanda, K. & Hashizume, K. (1992) Factors causing differences in force output among motor units in the cat medialis gastrocnemius muscle. *J Physiol,* Vol. 448, pp. 677-695.

Kandel, ER., Schwartz, JH. & Jessel, TM. (1995). Essentials of neural science and behaviour. New York, USA: McGraw-Hill.

Keenan, KG. & Valero-Cuevas, FJ. (2007) Experimentally valid predictions of muscle force and EMG in models of motor-unit function are most sensitive to neural properties. *J Neurophysiol,* Vol. 98, pp. 1581-1590.

Keenan, KG., Farina, D., Merletti, R. & Enoka, RM. (2006) Influence of motor unit properties on the size of the simulated evoked surface EMG potential. *Exp Brain Res,* Vol. 169, pp. 37-49.

Kernell, D., Eerbeek, O. & Verhey, BA. (1983) Motor unit categorization on basis of contractile properties: an experimental analysis of the composition of the cat's muscle peroneus longus. *Exp Brain Res,* Vol. 50, pp. 211-219.

Kim , MS., Masakado, Y., Tomita, Y., Chino, N., Pae, YS., Lee, KE. (2001). Synchornization of single motor units during voluntary contractions in the upper and lower extremities. *Clin Neurophisiol.* Vol. 112. pp. 1243-1249.

Kleine, BU, Stegemean, DF., Mund, D. & Anders, C. (2001). Influence of motorneuron firing synchronization on SEMG characteristics in dependence to electrode position. *J. Appl Physiol.* Vol. 91, pp 1588-1599.

Kossev, A., Chistova, P. (1998). Discharge pattern of human motor units during dynamic concentric and eccentric contractions. *Electroenceph Clin Neurophysiol,* Vol. 109, pp. 345-255.

Li, B.; Xu, Y. & Choi, J. (1996). Applying Machine Learning Techniques, *Proceedings of ASME 2010 4th International Conference on Energy Sustainability,* pp. 14-17, ISBN 842-6508-23-3, Phoenix, Arizona, USA, May 17-22, 2010

Lieber, RL. (2010). Skeletal muscle structure, function, and plasticity, Baltimore, MD: Lippincott Williams & Wilkins.

Lima, P.; Bonarini, A. & Mataric, M. (2004). *Application of Machine Learning,* InTech, ISBN 978-953-7619-34-3, Vienna, Austria

Lorente de No, R. (1947). Analysis of the distribution of action currents of nerve in volume conductors. Studies from the *Rockefeller Inst. Med. Res.,* Vol. 132, pp. 384-485.

Lowery, M., Stoykov, NS., Dewald, JPA. & Kuiken, TA. (2004). Volume conduction in an anatomically based surface EMG model. *IEEE Trans Biomed Eng,* Vol. 51, pp. 2138-2147.

Lowery, M., Stoykov, NS., Taflove, A. & Kuiken, TA. A multiple-layer finite-element model of the surface EMG signal. *IEEE Trans Biomed Eng,* Vol. 49, pp. 446-454.

Ludin, H. (1973). Action potentials of normal and dystrophic human muscle fibers. In: *New development in electromyography and clinical neurophysiology,* pp. 400–406, Desmedt JE, Basel: Karger.

Matthews, PB. (1996). Relationship of firing intervals of human motor units to the trajectory of post-spike afterhypolarization and synaptic noise. *J. Physiol.*Vol. 492, pp 597-628.

McGill, KC., (2004). Surface electromyographic signal modelling. *Med Biol Eng Compt.* Vol. 42, pp. 446–454.

McGill, KC., Lateva, ZC., & Xiao, S. (2001). A model of the muscle action potential for describing the leading edge, terminal wave, and slow afterwave. *IEEE Trans Biomed Eng,* Vol. 48, pp. 1357–1365.

McIntosh, BR., Gardiner, PF. & McComas, AJ. (2006) *Skeletal muscle: form and function.* Human Kinetics, 2nd edition.

Merletti, R. & Parker, PA. (2004). Electromyography: physiology, engineering and noninvasive applications. New Jersey, USA: IEEE Press-John Wiley and Sons.

Merletti, R., Lo Conte, L., Avignone & Gugielminotti, P. (1999). Modeling of surface myoelectric signals-Part I: model implementation. *IEEE Trans Biomed Eng,* Vol. 46, pp. 810-820.

Mesin, L. (2008) Simulation of surface EMG signals for a multilayer volume conductor with a superficial bone or blood vessel. *IEEE Trans Biomed Eng*, Vol. 55, pp. 1647-1657.

Mesin, L., Farina, D. (2004). Simulation of surface EMG signals generated by muscle tissues with inhomogeneity due to fiber pinnation. *IEEE Trans Biomed Eng*, Vol. 51, pp. 1521-1529.

Miller-Larsson, A. (1980) A model of spatial distribution of muscle fibers of a motor unit in normal human limb muscles. *Electroencephalogr Clin Neurophysiol*, Vol. 20, pp. 281-298.

Milner-Brown, HS., Stein RB., & Yemm, R., (1973). Changes in firing rate of human motor units during linearly changing voluntary contractions. *J. Physiol. Lond.* Vol. 230, pp 371-390.

Monster, AW., Chan, H (1977). Isometric force production by motor units of extensor digitorum communis muscle in man. *J. Neurophysiol.* Vol. 40, pp 1432-1443.

Nandedkar, S. & Stålberg, E (1983) Simulation of single muscle fiber action potentials. *Med Biol Eng Comput*, Vol. 21, pp. 158-165.

Nandedkar, S., & Stalberg, E. (1983). Simulation of Macro EMG motor unit action potentials. *EEG Clin Neurophysiol*, Vol. 56, pp. 52–62.

Nandedkar, SD., Sanders, DB, Stålberg, EV. & Andreassen, S. (1988) Simulation of concentric needle EMG motor unit action potentials. *Muscle Nerve*, Vol. 11, pp. 151-159.

Nandedkar S.D., Sanders D.B., (1989). Simulation of myopathic motor unit action potentials. Muscle and Nerve 12, pp. 197-202.

Navallas & Stålberg (2009) Studying motor end-plate topography by means of scanning-electromyography. *Clin Neurphysiol*, Vol. 120, pp. 1335-1341.

Navallas, J., Malanda, A., Gila, L., Rodríguez, J. & Rodríguez, I. (2009a) Mathematical analysis of a muscle architecture model. *Math Biosci*, Vol. 217, pp. 64-76.

Navallas, J., Malanda, A., Gila, L., Rodríguez, J. & Rodríguez, I. (2009b) Comparative evaluation of motor unit architecture models. *Med Biol Eng Comput*, Vol. 47, pp. 1131-1142.

Navallas, J., Malanda, A., Gila, L., Rodríguez, J. & Rodríguez, I. (2010) A muscle architecture model offering control over motor unit fiber density distributions. *Med Biol Eng Comput*, Vol. 48, pp. 875-886.

Plonsey, R. (1974). The active fiber in a volume conductor. *IEEE Trans Biomed Eng*, Vol. 21, pp. 371–381.

Plonsey, R., &Barr RC. (2000). Bioelectricity. A quantitative approach, New York, USA: Kluwer Academic.

Rodríguez J, Navallas J, Gila L, Latasa I & Malanda A. (2012). Effects of changes in the shape of the intracellular action potential on the peak-to-peak ratio of single muscle fibre potentials. *J Electromyogr Kinesiol*. Vol. 22(1). pp. 88-97.

Rodriguez, J., Malanda, A., Gila, L., Rodríguez, I., & Navallas, J. (2011). Estimating the duration of intracellular action potentials in muscle fibres from single-fibre extracellular potentials. *J Neurosci Meth*, Vol. 197, pp. 221:230.

Roeleveld, K., Block, J.H., Stegeman, D.F. & Van Oosterom, A. (1997). Volume conductor models for surface EMG; confrontation with measurements. *J Electromyogr Kinesiol*. Vol. 7. pp. 221-232.

Schnetzer, MA., Ruegg, DG., Baltensperger, R. & Gabriel, JP. (2001) Three-dimensional model of a muscle and simulation of its surface EMG. *Proceedings of the 23rd Annual International Conference of the IEEE EMBS*, Vol. 2, pp. 1038-1043.

Sears, TA., & Stagg, D. (1976). Short term synchronization of intercostal motoneurone activity. *J. Physiol.* Vol. 263, pp 357-381.

Semmler, J.G., Nordstrom, MA., Wallace CJ. (1997). Relationship between motor unit short-term synchornization and common drive in human first dorsal interosseous muscle. *Brain Research.* Vol. 767. pp. 314-320.

Shenhav, R. & Gath, I. (1986) Simulation of the spatial distribution of muscle fibers in human muscle. *Comput Methods Programs Biomed*, Vol. 23, pp.3-9.

Siegwart, R. (2001). Indirect Manipulation of a Sphere on a Flat Disk Using Force Information. *International Journal of Advanced Robotic Systems*, Vol.6, No.4, (December 2009), pp. 12-16, ISSN 1729-8806

Stålberg, E. & Antoni, L. (1980) Electrophysiological cross section of the motor unit. *J Neurol Neurosurg Psychiatr*, Vol. 43, pp. 464-474.

Stålberg, E. & Karlsson, L. (2001) Simulation of the normal concentric needle electromyogram by using a muscle model. *Clin Neurophysiol*, Vol. 112, pp. 464-471.

Stalberg E., Karlsson, L. (2001). Simulation of EMG in pathological situations. Clinical Neurophysiology 112 pp. 869-878.

Stålberg, E. (1966) Propagation velocity in human muscle fibres in situ. *Acta Physiol Scand*, Vol. 70, suppl. 287, pp. 1-112.

Stålberg, E., & Trontelj J. (1979). Single fibre electromyography. Old Woking, UK: Raven Press.

Stålberg, E., & Trontelj J. (1992). Clinical neurophysiology: the motor unit in myopathy. In: *Handbook of clinical neurology*, pp. 49 – 84, Rowland LP. New York: Elsevier.

Stashuk, DW. (1993) Simulation of electromyographic signals. *J Electromyogr Kinesiol*, Vol. 3, pp. 157-173.

Van der Linden, S. (June 2010). Integrating Wind Turbine Generators (WTG's) with Energy Storage, In: Wind Power, 17.06.2010, Available from

Wakeling, JM. (2009). Patterns of motor recruitment can be determined by using surface EMG. J Electromyogr Kinesiol. Vol. 19. pp. 199-207.

Westgaard R.H., De Luca J.C., (1999). Motor unit substitution in long duration contractions of the human trapezius muscle. J Neurophysiol 82, pp. 501-504.

Wilson, F., MacLeod, A., & Barker, P. (1933). The distribution of the action currents produced by heart muscle and other excitable tissues immersed in extensive conducting media. *J Gen Physical*, Vol. 16, pp. 423–456.

Yao, W., Fugglevand, AJ., Enoka, RM. (2000). Motor unit synchronization increases EMG amplitude and decreases force steadiness of simulated contractions. *J. Neurophysiol.* Vol. 83, pp 441-452.

Zhou, P. & Rymer, WZ. (2004). Factors governing the form of relationship between muscle force and the EMG: a simulation study. *J. Neurophysiol.* Vol. 92, pp 2878-2886.

# Chapter 2

# Modelling of Transcranial Magnetic Stimulation in One-Year Follow-Up Study of Patients with Minor Ischaemic Stroke

Penka A. Atanassova, Nedka T. Chalakova and Borislav D. Dimitrov

Additional information is available at the end of the chapter

## 1. Introduction

Since its commercial advent in 1985, transcranial magnetic stimulation (TMS), a technique for stimulating neurons in the cerebral cortex through the scalp, safely and with minimal discomfort, has captured the imaginations of scientists, clinicians and lay observers [Wassermann et al, 2012]. Initially a laboratory tool for neurophysiologists studying the human motor system, TMS now has a growing list of applications in clinical and basic neuroscience. At cortical level, the abnormal amplitudes of the motor evoked potentials (MEP) may be due to the damage of the motoneurons themselves; as well as to their reduced capacity for repetitive excitation; deficit of the intracortical synaptic transmission (transfer); activation of motoneuron inhibitors, etc. At subcortical level the causes may be demyelinization, remyelinization, activation of the long-latent corticofugal fibres, axonal damage, etc. [Komori et al, 1993].

The human brain possesses a remarkable ability to adapt in response to changing anatomical (e.g., aging) or environmental modifications. This form of neuroplasticity is important at all stages of life but is critical in neurological disorders such as amblyopia and stroke [Sharma, 2012]. When MEP are obtained in the acute phase of stroke, the functional recovery of the motor deficit, as a rule, is to occur [Nowak et al, 2010; Dimyan, 2010]. The initially registered normal MEP amplitudes have a predictive value in the view of the long-term functional outcome [Stinear, 2010; Dimyan et al, 2010;].

The TMS approach was also used in the investigation of patients with lacunar strokes. The central motor conduction time (CMCT) and the threshold intensities for eliciting MEPs in the relaxed muscles were significantly increased on the affected side. MEP amplitude abnormalities were related to pyramidal signs (though they could be observed also in a patient without any motor impairment) and occurred independently of a specific clinical picture or a radiologically confirmed lacunar lesion [Abbruzzese et al, 1991; Hufnagel et al, 1990]. Earlier studies have shown that during the acute phase of the minor ischaemic stroke (MIS), MEP amplitudes can be registered in all investigated patients [Hadjipetrova et al, 1993]. To note, the increases in the latency of the M-response and CMCT have prognostic significance for early assessment of the outcome of ischaemic stroke [Stulin et al, 2003]. Earlier studies by Ferbert and collaborators [1992] have indicated that the MEP amplitudes are a more sensitive marker for the sublclinical damage of the pyramidal tract than CMCT. A significant correlation has also been reported among the recovery of muscle strength and the amplitude of MEP [Palliyath, 2000].

The aim of this study was to perform a *post-hoc* analysis of one-year follow-up data from 40 patients with MIS and to: (i) investigate the central motor conduction time (CMCT) and the amplitude of the motor evoked potential (MEP) during the acute phase of MIS; (ii) provide evidence for a subclinical damage of the pyramidal tract; and (iii) model and predict the outcome measures at month 12 after MIS as based on earlier changes in the acute phase.

## 2. Methods

### 2.1. Patient selection, diagnosis, data collection, and main characteristics

The Plovdiv project included hospital-based incident cases of patients with minor ischaemic stroke (MIS) that were followed for 12 months to determine the estimates of central motor conduction time (CMCT) and amplitudes of motor evoked potential (MEP) and their changes and correlations over time.

This is a *post-hoc* analysis and modelling study. The patient population has been described in more detail earlier [Atanassova, 1998; Atanasova & Vukov, 1998; Atanassova, Voukov & Tchalakova, 2002; Atanassova, Chalakova & Dimitrov, 2008a]. In particular, patients with cerebrovascular disease had been hospitalized in the Clinic of Cerebrovascular Diseases (Plovdiv Healthcare Region) and 56 consecutive patients with MIS were subjected to screening. All screened, eligible patients with MIS as an initial index event who provided a written, informed consent in accordance with the Declaration of Helsinki guidelines at discharge were immediately enrolled. During the lag interval from the index event until discharge (i.e., during the hospital stay), no vascular events were observed among the 56 screened eligible patients. Of these eligible patients, 54 patients (96.4%) provided written, informed consent and were included in the current follow-up study. The other 2 eligible patients did not provide informed consent at discharge and were not enrolled (**Figure 1**). Further, till month 12, a total of 14 patients were excluded or lost to follow-up and could not provide data on the outcome, therefore, 40 patients were subjected to statistical analyses and modelling in this study. The inclusion criteria were: patients with first MIS, age > 40 years and residence in Plovdiv for at least three months before identification and enrolment [Atanassova, Chalakova & Dimitrov, 2008a]. All evaluations were performed at Medical University Hospital of Plovdiv, Bulgaria. The University Ethical Committee approved the study protocol.

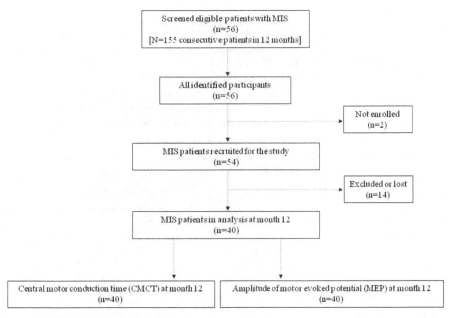

**Figure 1.** CONSORT flow-chart of study screening, enrolment and analysis.

Data were collected by instructed physicians and clinical (physical and neurological) examinations were conducted by study neurologists [Atanassova, Chalakova & Dimitrov, 2008a]. The assessments covered: hypertension, diabetes, dyslipidaemia, peripheral vascular disease, cardiac conditions, cigarette smoking, educational background, etc.

Initial stroke severity was assessed using the modified Rankin Scale [Bamford et al, 1990]. MIS diagnostic evaluations included CT or MRI of the brain and ultrasound evaluation and/or trans-thoracic or trans-oesophageal echocardiogram, as appropriate. A panel of stroke neurologists assessed every CV events subtype using standard diagnostic criteria and all available information for each patient. For this study, *MIS* was defined as a minor stroke if the score on the modified Rankin Scale was 1 at the first evaluation, or if the score was 0 or 1 at one-month follow-up (i.e., no symptoms, or minor symptoms that did not interfere with normal lifestyle) [Atanassova, 1998; Atanasova & Vukov, 1998; Atanassova, Voukov & Tchalakova, 2002]. In particular, acute onset was observed in 11 patients (20.4%). Extra-cranial ultrasound findings were recorded in 11 patients (20.4%). The main characteristics of the initial study cohort were as follows: 37 men (68.5%) and 17 women (31.5%), with male predominance in CV events (n=8 men) but with similar ages of 61.1±12.6 years in patients with CVE versus 62.2±9.2 years in patients without CVE (p>0.05). The mean follow-up time was 11.1±2.4 months with mean time to CV events of 5.8±2.7 months. For the purpose of this study, all MIS patients with subsequent stroke (n=8) as defined above, were excluded from the analysis.

## 2.1.1. Assessment of outcomes

The main outcome was defined as estimates of central motor conduction time (CMCT) and amplitudes of motor evoked potential (MEP) at month 12. We performed transcranial magnetic stimulation by MAGSTIM 200 after MIS (day 7 in month 1, month 3, and month 12) on the motor cerebral cortex bilaterally and on C7 with consecutive conduction of MEPs by surface electrodes from isometrically slightly contracted muscle *abductor policis brevis*. All measurements were taken as related to the symptomatic and asymptomatic hemispheres and differences between them were also analysed (Table 1). Normal values from 30 healthy subjects were also obtained for reference purposes.

| Outcome parameters in MIS patients (n=40 patients) | Symptomatic hemisphere (n=40 cases*) | Asymptomatic hemisphere (n=40 cases*) | p-value |
|---|---|---|---|
| Central motor conduction time (CMCT) *[ms]* | | | |
| at Month 1 (day 7) | 9.147 ± 1.862 | 7.550 ± 1.465 | <0.05 |
| at Month 3 | 8.038 ± 1.392 | 7.135 ± 1.052 | <0.05 |
| at Month 12 | 10.720 ± 1.831 | 8.550 ± 1.497 | <0.05 |
| Amplitude of motor evoked potential (MEP) *[mV]* | | | |
| at Month 1 (day 7) | 6.083 ± 1.882 | 8.963 ± 1.925 | <0.05 |
| at Month 3 | 7.293 ± 1.876 | 10.350 ± 2.160 | <0.05 |
| at Month 12 | 7.290 ± 1.757 | 9.880 ± 1.986 | <0.05 |

Notes: *Number of cases (measurements) in the MIS patients with TMS values; Data are mean ± standard deviation; °Difference at $p<0.05$ is considered statistically significant. Abbreviations: MIS, minor ischaemic stroke.

**Table 1.** Main outcomes of TMS in 40 MIS patients, followed prospectively for 12 months, as measured according to the existing symptomatics (symptomatic or asymptomatic hemisphere)

As secondary outcomes, the changes from month 1 onwards, as well as the correlations between the estimates, were also analysed. The role of the symptomatics (i.e., measures for symptomatic or asymptomatic hemisphere) as a predictor of the main outcome estimates at month 12, was also investigated. The presence/absence of non-fatal or fatal CV event after MIS was considered for the diagnosis of the MIS patients with a subsequent stroke, who were to be excluded from the analyses. Thus, two2 sub-categories for each secondary outcome were established as events classification: (i) non-fatal CVE; (ii) fatal CVE. Strict evaluations were conducted in 4 visits (at baseline, at month 1, month 3 and month 12), with telephone interview every other month, till month 12. Every evaluation was carried-out by contact with the patient, family member, or caregiver. Information was collected by somatic examination, inter-current symptoms, illness or hospitalization. The in-person visits were conducted at our clinic and included measuring vital signs, physical and neurological examination. A registry reporting system was used to identify study participants who experienced nonfatal or fatal vascular events, related hospitalization or death (vascular or nonvascular death). All records were reviewed for all outcome events, including death, and have been maintained. All outcome events were reviewed by a neurology specialist. Non-fatal strokes were validated by a study neurologist, and all deaths were to be validated, as well. Deaths were to be classified using death certificates and medical records.

Death as an eventual fatal outcome was defined as to be considered as due to stroke if there was clear documentation of a stroke from the death certificate or hospital records; deaths that would have occurred more than 30 days after the initial accident (i.e., secondary CV event) had to be considered related to the event on the grounds of a clinical judgment that relied on a clearly documented relationship to the stroke or its complications to the point of death in the medical records. Following the ascertainment procedures, all above mentioned death notifications, certificates, and autopsy protocols for all cases of death had to be collected and reviewed individually, especially for patients who died outside the hospital. In cases in which it was difficult to determine whether death was due to stroke, consensus was reached after discussion using the best available information.

## 2.2. Sample size, data elaboration and statistical analyses

### 2.2.1. Sample size estimation

The sample size of the initial follow-up cohort of 56 patients to be screened was calculated on the basis of the expected number of CV events, as described previously in more detail [Atanassova, Chalakova & Dimitrov, 2008a]. Having assumed a theoretical distribution from 0 to 50% for the non-events and based on the 3-year cumulative incidence of 24.5% for cerebrovascular events in MIS patients [Atanassova, Chalakova & Dimitrov, 2008b], 8.16% of CV events were to be expected in 12 months. Thus, it had been estimated that to give the study >95% power to detect such minimum event rate as statistically significant at p<0.05, 51 patients had to be included and analysed. A preliminary estimate of the prevalence of MIS patients that would satisfy the inclusion/exclusion criteria from all those referred to the Clinic of Cerebrovascular Diseases yearly had indicated that 56 patients with MIS had to be identified throughout a screening period of about 12 months (estimated maximum 10% drop-out). Given the pilot nature of the probabilistic modelling of the estimates and derivation of predictions at month 12 for both studied parameters (CMCT and MEP), no further sample size calculations were performed.

### 2.2.2. Data elaboration and statistical analyses

The main endpoint for both the central motor conduction time and amplitudes of motor evoked potentials was considered as an estimated mean (± standard deviation, S.D.) at month 12 (**Table 1**). Two other interim measures of the outcomes were also taken (at month 1 and month 3). A test for normality of distributions (Shapiro-Wilk test) was applied. The differences were analysed by two-tailed paired parametric (t-test, etc.) or non-parametric (Wilcoxon signed-rank) tests at p<0.05, as appropriate, as well as repeated-measures

ANOVA (general linear models) in the view of the symptomatic and asymptomatic hemispheres (**Figure 2 & Figure 3**). As appropriate, parametric and non-parametric correlations between CMCT and MEP at various times were also performed.

Parametric regression modelling was used to analyse the data and develop models to predict the outcomes at month 12 (**Table 2**). The significant relationships were later explored and confirmed by probabilistic artificial neural network (ANN) modelling, irrespectively of usual statistical constraints (**Figures 4 & Figure 5**). The stopping rule of learning was assumed when a state of maximum overall correctness of prediction with minimum average learning error was reached [Sarle, 1997]. The p-values less than 0.05 were considered statistically significant. The specialised software packages for statistical (SPSS ver.18) and probabilistic modelling (EasyNN ver.6.0i) were used.

## 3. Results

### 3.1. Descriptive statistics and basic comparisons

The recruited patient cohort consisted of 54 patients (37 males and 17 females), mean age of 62 years (SD 9.6). The neurological deficit by the Rankin's scale was assess at mRs=1 (37 patients), mRs=2 (16 patients) and mRs=3 (1 patient). Most frequent minor ischaemic strokes occurred in the left carotid system (53.7%), right carotid system (31.4%), both systems (9.3%) as well as in the vertebrobasilar system (5.6%). Most frequently observed are the syndromes of the middle cerebral artery (hemiparesis and involvement of VII and XII cranial nerves), aphasias after a damage of the dominant hemisphere, upper monoparesis and motor aphasia, etc. In particular, during the mean follow-up of 11.1±2.4 months, 8 secondary CV events (14.8%) were observed only in males within a mean period of 5.8±2.7 months. No difference in the age of patients with CV event (61.1±12.6 years) vs. those without (62.1±9.6 years) was found (p>0.05). The one-year risk for CVE was ≈15% (95%CI 7.1÷27.7%). The other main demographic and clinical parameters of the initial cohort of 54 patients were reported in a more detail earlier [Atanassova, Chalakova & Dimitrov, 2008a].

The main results are summarized in Table 1. Although the distributions of CMCT at month 12 in the asymptomatic hemisphere and MEP at month 1 in the symptomatic one were slightly skewed, two tendencies could be clearly observed. While there is clearly a difference in the TMS measures according to the existing symptomatics (i.e., symptomatic or asymptomatic hemisphere), the first one is an increase of CMCT over time with higher values in the symptomatic hemisphere, while the second one is again an increase of MEP over time, but the higher values this time are observed in the asymptomatic hemisphere (p<0.05).

An interesting pattern is, however, that while CMCT first decreased from month 1 to month 3 and then increased (Figure 2), the MEP amplitude, in parallel but opposite, increased in month 3 and then decreased slightly in month 12 (Figure 3). In particular, there was a significant change over time (p<0.001) in CMCT and a multivariate, combined effect of symptomatics and time (grand mean 8.523 ms, 95%CI 8.240-8.805, p=0.01). Notably, there was a statistically significant difference (adjusted for the baseline values at month 1) between the estimated marginal means of CMCT in the symptomatic (10.717 ms, 95%CI 10.191-11.244) and asymptomatic (8.023 ms, 95%CI 8.023-9.077) hemispheres (Figure 2).

There was a significant increase over time (p<0.001) in MEP amplitude, however, the multivariate, combined effect of symptomatics and time was not significant (grand mean 8.310 mV, 95%CI 7.922-8.697, p=0.309). Certainly, there was a statistically significant difference between the estimated marginal means of MEP amplitude in the symptomatic (6.888 mV, 95%CI 6.340-7.437) and asymptomatic (9.731 mV, 95%CI 9.182-10.279) hemispheres, but this was observed since month 1 and continued as such till month 12 (Figure 3).

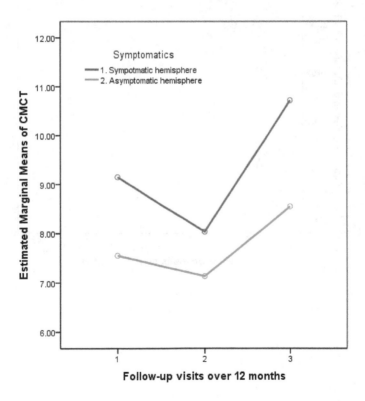

**Figure 2.** General linear modelling (repeated ANOVA) of CMCT changes from month 1 till month 12

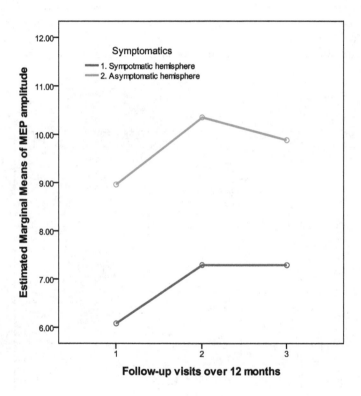

**Figure 3.** General linear modelling (repeated ANOVA) of MEP amplitude changes from month 1 till month 12

Since these changes appeared to be parallel, we tested also the correlations between the
measurements of TMS parameters at different months. In particular, there was a weak
inverse, but significant correlations between CMCT and MEP (Spearman's Rho=-0.45-0.46,
p<0.05). Notably, the highest positive correlations were observed between CMCT at month 1
and the following months (0.60-0.81, p<0.05) as well as between MEP at month 1 and the
following months (0.78-0.87, p<0.05). The latter relationships provided the opportunity to
model and predict the outcome at month 12 in the two TMS parameters.

## 3.2. Statistical and probabilistic modelling of the outcome at 12 months

The parametric regression modelling indicated that the CMCT outcome at month 12 can be
predicted by the initial values at month 1 and whether or not these have been observed in
the symptomatic or asymptomatic hemisphere (Fmodel=33.323, p<0.001, Table 2). The same
is valid for the MEP amplitude outcome at month 12 (Fmodel=55.0.09, p<0.001, Table 2),
although the role of the symptomatic as a predictor is with a marginal statistical significance
(p=0.051).

| Outcome parameters in 40 MIS patients | Independent variables | Standardized coefficient β* | p-value |
|---|---|---|---|
| Central motor conduction time at month 12 | CMCT at month 1 | 0.448 | <0.001 |
| | Symptomatics | -0.354 | <0.001 |
| Amplitude of motor evoked potential at month 12 | Amplitude of MEP at month 1 | 0.642 | <0.001 |
| | Symptomatics | 0.183 | 0.051 |

Notes: *The predictor "symptomatics" is a categorical variable referring to the particular hemisphere, with two
categories: symptomatic and asymptomatic. The constants, unstandardized coefficients β and their standards errors
are available from the authors upon request. Abbreviations: TMS, transcranial magnetic stimulation; CMCT, central
motor conduction time; MEP, motor evoked potential.

**Table 2.** Parametric regression modelling to predict the TMS outcomes in 40 patients at month 12

The above relationships were further investigated by a probabilistic modelling, employing
artificial neural network (ANN) methodology, which has not the usual constrains of a
parametric regression analyses (Figure 4 & Figure 5). The ANN for modelling and
predicting CMCT at month 12 contained 9 nodes with 2 hidden layers, with two potential
predictors: CMCT at month 1 and symptomatics (symptomatic or asymptomatic
hemisphere) (Fig. 4). The structure for predicting the resulting outcome node was obtained
when the average error decreased below the target value of 0.049.

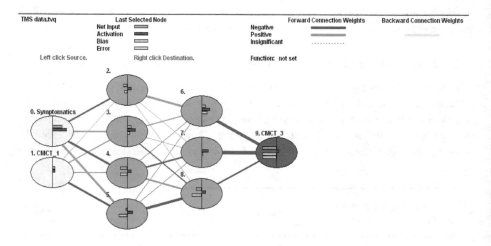

Legend: Yellow circles (No.0–1) on the left indicate 2 input variables. The magenta circle (No.9) on the right is the output variable (outcome). The nodes of two hidden layers are grouped vertically and coloured in cyan: hidden layer 1 (nodes No.2–5); hidden layer 2 (nodes No.6–8). ANN nodes description: Each node contains small bar charts indicating the basic functional parameters – net input (cyan bar), activation (magenta bar), bias (orange bar) and error (yellow bar). The hidden nodes are connected by lines, showing the type and strength of weights: the red and green lines indicate negative and positive weights, respectively. The thicker the line is, the heavier the weight.

**Figure 4.** Artificial neural network trained with 40 patients to predict the CMCT outcome at month 12

The modelling confirmed the finding from the parametric regression analysis ($\beta$=0.448, Table 2) for a slightly higher relative (predictive) importance of the CMCT at month 1 (0.301) than symptomatics ($\beta$=-0.354, relative importance = 0.290, not shown).

The ANN for modelling and predicting MEP at month 12 contained 16 nodes with 2 hidden layers, with two potential predictors: MEP at month 1 and symptomatics (symptomatic or asymptomatic hemisphere) (Fig. 5). The structure for predicting the resulting outcome node was obtained when the average error decrease below the target value of 0.049. The modelling confirmed the finding from the parametric regression analysis ($\beta$=0.642, Table 2) for a quite higher relative (predictive) importance of the MEP at month 1 (relative importance = 230.19) than symptomatics ($\beta$=0.183, relative importance = 62.06, not shown).

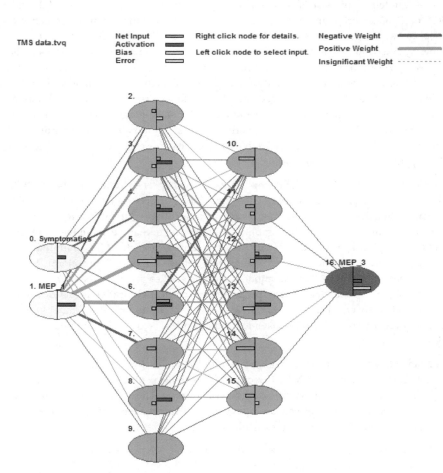

Legend: Yellow circles (No.0–1) on the left indicate 2 input variables. The magenta circle (No.16) on the right is the output variable (outcome). The nodes of two hidden layers are grouped vertically and coloured in cyan: hidden layer 1 (nodes No.2–9); hidden layer 2 (nodes No.10–15). ANN nodes description: Each node contains small bar charts indicating the basic functional parameters – net input (cyan bar), activation (magenta bar), bias (orange bar) and error (yellow bar). The hidden nodes are connected by lines, showing the type and strength of weights: the red and green lines indicate negative and positive weights, respectively. The thicker the line is, the heavier the weight.

**Figure 5.** Artificial neural network trained with 40 patients to predict the MEP amplitude outcome at month 12

## 4. Discussion

The one-year follow-up established a statistically significant dynamics in the MEP and CMCT outcomes. During the acute phase of the ischaemic stroke in the symptomatic hemisphere we found prolonged CMCT and reduced MEP amplitudes, similar to the findings by other authors [Segura et al, 1990]. When abnormal MEP amplitude is found, it is most likely the case of mainly functional disturbances of the pyramidal tract conduction, with a pathogenesis due to the acute disorder of cerebral circulation [Braune et al, 1996]. This may probably explain the prolonged latencies of MEP and reduced MEP amplitudes in the asymptomatic hemisphere. The decrease of the CMCT and the significant increase of the MEP amplitude (without reaching the normal values) at month 3, an according to Hadjipetrova et al [1993] – even at the 20-th day after the index event – could be explained with temporary functional compensation after MIS.

According to some authors, the MEP amplitudes are a more sensitive marker than CMCT in the view of assessing the damage of the corticospinal tracts as a result of the brain ischaemia. After the acute phase, there might be a facillitation at cortical level, which could allow an increase in the MEP amplitude and may eventually explain the increases in the MEP amplitude at month 3 in our patients. In particular, the MEP amplitudes in the asymptomatic hemisphere achieve the normal values at month 3 and month 12. In the same time, it is known that the minor ischaemic strokes are most likely of lacunar type (i.e., "deep", "subcortical"). The proportion of cortical clinical syndromes in our patients is relatively small and we could hypothesize that the abnormal MEP amplitudes might be present also in distant ischaemic lesion as it was shown earlier [Laloux et al, 1991].

At month 12, even in patients without neurological deficit and without recurrent cerebrovascular accidents, the CMCT is increased in both hemispheres. MEP amplitudes at month 12 are also reduced in the view of the normal values. These later changes are most likely due to the appearance of new asymptomatic structural changes of the corticospinal tracts during the progression of cerebrovascular disease.

Last but not least, following the revealed correlations, we were also able to create predictive models for the outcomes at month 12. For both the CMCT and MEP amplitude, the regression models were based on the initial measures at month 1 and symptomatics (i.e., pertaining to symptomatic or asymptomatic hemisphere). We confirmed our results further by using such probabilistic approach as artificial neural networks modelling. ANN proved to be very useful in the current analysis as it allowed us to assess the role of potential predictors of CMCT and MEP at month 12 as continuous outcomes, without the possible constraints of parametric models (e.g., normal distribution of the outcome, etc.). To note, ANN had been successfully used in other medical fields [Mecocci, 2002; Grossi, 2011; Azarkhish et al, 2012; etc.] and, in neurology, in particular [Mecocci, 2002; Shanthi et al, 2009; for a recent overview see Atanassova & Dimitrov, 2011].

## 5. Conclusions

This *post-hoc* analysis of one-year follow-up clinical trial data, obtained in 40 patients with minor ischaemic stroke, but without neurological deficit or recurrent cerebrovascular incidents, established a statistically significant dynamics in the MEP and CMCT outcomes after transcranial magnetic stimulation. During the acute phase of the ischaemic stroke (at day 7 in month 1) we performed an initial measurement on the motor cerebral cortex bilaterally and on C7 with consecutive conduction of MEPs by surface electrodes from isometrically slightly contracted muscle *abductor policis brevis* and found prolonged CMCT and reduced MEP amplitudes in the symptomatic hemisphere. By following consecutive measurements at the end of month 3 and month 12, we revealed that the CMCT was increased in both hemispheres and MEP amplitudes were reduced, thus both remaining with abnormal values. At the interim measurement, CMCT were shorter but still abnormal in both hemispheres while the MEP amplitudes were lower, mostly in the symptomatic hemisphere. The changes at the end of the follow-up are most likely due to the appearance of new asymptomatic structural changes of the corticospinal tracts during the progression of the cerebrovascular disease.

We observed a parallel dynamics and found correlations between CMCT and MEP at various times, preserving a significant asymmetry among the two hemisepheres. There was a statistically significant correlation between the initial values of CMCT and MEP and the outcome measurements at month 12. The parametric regression modelling indicated that CMCT outcomes at month 12 can be predicted by the initial values at month 1 and whether or not these have been observed in the symptomatic or asymptomatic hemisphere. The same is valid for the MEP amplitude outcomes at month 12, although the role of the symptomatics as a predictor is with a marginal statistical significance. The probabilistic ANN modelling confirmed the role of early CMCT (month 1) and hemisphere symptomatics in predicting the outcome at month 12. Given the dynamics of CMCT and MEP changes, we could postulate that cerebrovascular disease progression post-MIS may have most likely determined the subclinical damage of the pyramidal tract and its underlying mechanisms.

## 6. Future directions

Early MEP recordings in acute stroke patients provide valid prognostic information; they may become more useful for specific treatment decisions than presently available MRI surrogate parameters (Wohrle, 2004). The presence of MEP and disruption of the corticospinal tract on diffusion tensor tractography at the early stage of corona radiata infarct are indicative of a high probability of good and poor motor outcome at the chronic stage, respectively. We would suggest that further studies involving more parameters for TMS are warranted (Kwon, 2011).

## Author details

Penka A. Atanassova and Nedka T. Chalakova
*Department of Neurology; Medical University, Plovdiv, Bulgaria*

Borislav D. Dimitrov

*Department of General Practice, Division of Population Health Sciences,*
*Royal College of Surgeons in Ireland, Dublin, Republic of Ireland*

*Academic Unit of Primary Care and Population Sciences,*
*University of Southampton, Southampton, United Kingdom*

# 7. References

Abbruzzese G, Morena M, Dall'Agata D et al (1991). Motor evoked potentials (MEP) in lacunar syndromes. *Electroencephalography & Clinical Neurophysiology,* 81, 202-208.

Azarkhish I, Raoufy MR, Gharibzadeh S (2012). Artificial intelligence models for predicting iron deficiency anaemia and iron serum level based on accessible laboratory data. *Journal of Medical Systems,* 36(3), 2057-2061.

Atanasova P, Vukov M (1998). Probability for arising of a repeated vascular incident after the primary brain infarction, with a complete clinical repair. *Social Medicine,* 1, 19-20 (In Bulgarian with English Abstr)

Atanassova P (1998). *Clinical and ElectrophysiologicalvStudy of Patients with Minor Stroke,* D.M. Thesis, MU-Plovdiv, Bulgaria.

Atanassova PA, Dimitrov BD (2011). Recent advances and challenges in the application of artificial neural networks (ANN) in the neurological sciences: an overview. In: Kwon SJ, editor. *Artificial Neural Networks.* Hauppauge, NY, USA, Nova Publishers, pp.61-69.

Atanassova P, Voukov M, Tchalakova N (2002). Prediction models for probable subsequent cerebral events in patients with reversible ischaemic neurological deficit. *Cerebrovasc Dis,* 2, 10-15 (In Bulgarian with English Abstr)

Atanassova PA, Chalakova NT, Dimitrov BD (2008a). Diastolic blood pressure cut-off predicts major cerebrovascular events after minor ischaemic stroke: a post-hoc modelling study. *Central European Journal of Medicine,* 3, 430-437.

Atanassova PA, Chalakova NT, Dimitrov BD (2008b). Major vascular events after transient ischaemic attack and minor ischaemic stroke: post-hoc modelling of incidence dynamics. *Cerebrovascular Diseases,* 25, 225-233.

Bamford J, Sandercock P, Dennis M, Burn J, Warlow C (1990). A prospective study of acute cerebrovascular disease in the community: The Oxfordshire Community Stroke Project 1981-1986. Incidence, case fatality rates and overall outcome at one year of cerebral infarction, primary intracerebral and subarachnoid haemorrhage. *J Neurol Neurosurg Psychiatry,* 53, 16-22.

Braune HJ, Fritz C (1996). Assymetry of silent period evoked by transcranial magnetic stimulation in stroke patients. *Acta Neurologica Scandinavica,* 93, 168-174.

Dimyan MA, Cohen LG (2010). Contribution of transcranial magnetic stimulation to the understanding of functional recovery mechanisms after stroke. *Neurorehabil Neural Repair,* 24(2), 125-135.

Ferbert A, Vielhaber S, Meincke U et al (1992). Transcranial magnetic stimulation in pontine infarction:correlation to degree of paresis. *J Neurol Neurosurg & Psychiatry*, 55, 294-299.

Grossi E (2011). Artificial neural networks and predictive medicine: a revolutionary paradigm shift. In: *Artificial Neural Networks - Methodological Advances and Biomedical Applications*. (K Suzuki, ed), Rijeka, Croatia, InTech, pp.139-150.

Hadjipetrova E, Chalakova-Atanassova N, Vassileva T et al (1993). Pathogenetic aspects of clinicoelectrophysiological differentiation of transient cerebral circulation disorders terminating with a complete clinical recovery, *Folia Medica*, XXXV, 122, 37-44

Hufnagel, A, Jaeger M, Elger C (1990). Transcranial magnetic stimulation : specific facilitation of magnetic motor evoked potentials. *J Neurology*, 237, 416-419.

Komori, T, Brown W (1993). Central Electromyography. In: *Clinical Electromyography* (WF Brown, CF Bolton, eds.), Chapter 1, Butterworth-Hainemann, Ltd, Boston, USA.

Kwon YH, Son SM, Lee J, et al. (2011). Combined study of transcranial magnetic stimulation and diffusion tensor tractography for prediction of motor outcome in patients with corona radiata infarct. J Rehabil Med 2011; 43: 430–434

Laloux P, Brucher JM (1991). Lacunar infarcts due to cholesterol emboli. *Stroke*, 22, 1440-1444.

Mecocci P, Grossi E, Buscema M, Intraligi M, Savarè R, Rinaldi P, Cherubini A, Senin U (2002). Use of artificial networks in clinical trials: a pilot study to predict responsiveness to donepezil in Alzheimer's disease. *J Am Geriatr Soc*, 50(11), 1857-1860.

Nowak DA, Bösl K, Podubeckà J, Carey JR (2010). Noninvasive brain stimulation and motor recovery after stroke. *Restor Neurol Neurosci*, 28(4), 531-544.

Palliyath S (2000). Role of central conduction time and motor evoked response amplitude in predicting stroke outcome. *Electromyogr Clin Neurophysiol*, 40(5), 315-320.

Sarle WS, ed (1997). Neural Network FAQ, part 1 of 7. Introduction, periodic posting to the Usenet newsgroup comp.ai.neural-nets URL: ftp://ftp.sas.com/pub/neural/FAQ.html (last accessed on 29 Apr 2012).

Segura MJ, Gandolfo CN, Sica RE (1990). Central motor conduction in ischaemic and haemorrhagic cerebral lesions. *Electromyography & Clinical Neurophysiology*, 30, Suppl, 1, 41-45.

Shanthi D, Sahoo D, Saravanan N (2009). Designing an artificial neural network model for the prediction of thromboembolic stroke. *International Journals of Biometric and Bioinformatics*, 3(1), 10-18.

Sharma N, Cohen LG. (2012). Recovery of motor function after stroke. *Dev Psychobiol*, 54(3), 254-262.

Stinear C (2010). Prediction of recovery of motor function after stroke. *Lancet Neurol*, 9(12), 1228-1232.

Stulin ID, Savchenko AY, Smyalovskii VE, Musin RS, Stryuk GV, Priz IL, Bagir' VN, Semenova EN (2003). Use of transcranial magnetic stimulation with measurement of motor evoked potentials in the acute period of hemispheric ischemic stroke. *Neurosci Behav Physiol*, 33(5), 425-429.

Wassermann EM, Zimmermann T (2012). Transcranial magnetic brain stimulation: therapeutic promises and scientific gaps. *Pharmacol Ther*, 133(1), 98-107

Wöhrle JC, Behrens S, Mielke O, Hennerici MG (2004). Early motor evoked potentials in acute stroke: adjunctive measure to MRI for assessment of prognosis in acute stroke within 6 hours. *Cerebrovasc Dis*, 18(2), 130-134.

# Chapter 3

# Comparison by EMG of Running Barefoot and Running Shod

Begoña Gavilanes-Miranda, Juan J. Goiriena De Gandarias and
Gonzalo A. Garcia

Additional information is available at the end of the chapter

## 1. Introduction

Footwear is the "interface" between the locomotive system and the athlete's physical environment through which all the forces that act and react between the legs and the ground are transmitted.

According to Nigg (1986), the choice of footwear is based on the price, durability, comfort, colour, safety, weight, and performance; but, how footwear affects the human-ground interaction?

During jogging, running shoes have to reduce foot shock impact with the ground, to hold the foot, to control the pronation-supination, to direct the force at the time of propulsion for takeoff (Luethi & Stacoff 1987), and to increase efficiency.

Nowadays, more and more people practice sport, being jogging an activity common to many sports, besides being a sport specialty itself. Jogging is a complex activity requiring an exact timing of muscle activation and a precise control of movement. Many injuries occurred during jogging affect the musculoskeletal system: (1) tendonitis of: tibialis anterior, peroneus brevis, tibialis posterior, quadriceps, and Achilles tendon; (2) calcaneal apophysitis; (3) chronic syndromes: anterior and posterior compartments; (4) stress fractures; (5) plantar fasciitis; and (6) rupture of the hamstrings (Reber et al. 1993). Certain types of contractions may predispose the runner to a particular injury (Vaughan 1984).

The displacement speed is determined by the frequency and length of the stride. These variables are the result of the successful integration of many mechanical and neuromuscular processes.

The human body is a biological system that has many possibilities of action and reaction to external environmental influences. During the movement, the neuromuscular system is involved not only in the production of force to move the segments, but through different mechanisms sensory feedback is capable of reacting to small changes. Facilitation or reduction of these feedback mechanisms enable the human motor system for a wide variety of functions, such as: (1) control of the position and stiffness of joints, (2) shock absorption, (3) dynamic stability during the support, and (4) propulsion, facilitating that the involved muscles perform with suitable elastic and contractile characteristics (Gollhofer and Komi 1987).

During one cycle of jogging, lower extremities undergoes a phase of unipodal support (in which only of the feet is in contact with the ground), one of swinging, and two phases of flight (in which none of the feet are in contact with the ground): the first takes place before the swing phase and the second, after it. Support phase lasts less than 50% of the stride. Slocum & James (1968) divided the jogging stride in the following phases:

1.  Support (or stand) phase: begins when one foot contacts the ground and ends when the first finger of the same foot is no longer in contact with the ground. This phase can be subdivided into three: (1.a) impact phase; (1.b) phase of medium support or of absorption: time when the whole foot is resting on the ground; and (1.c) propulsion or push phase, which begins when the foot is lifted off the ground and ends when the toes leave the ground.
2.  Phase of no support or of recovery, which comprising three phases: (2.a) initial flight phase: begins when the first toe of the support foot is no longer in contact with the ground and ends when the heel of the contralateral foot (opposite one) touches the ground; (2.b) half swing phase: begins when the heel of the contralateral foot contacts the ground and ends when its first finger is no longer in contact with the ground; and (2.c) final flight phase: begins when the first finger of the opposite foot is no longer in contact with the ground and ends when the heel of the ipsilateral foot rests again on the floor.

Another way of dividing the non-phase support is as follows: period of follow-through (after leg takeoff, the hip stretches); forward period (the ipsilateral leg moves forward while the hip is flexed); and period of descend of the foot.

## 1.1. Movement of the joints

The displacement of the centre of gravity is due to the angular movement of the joints caused by the resultant of different forces: muscular force (caused by the neuromuscular system), ground reaction force, weight of the segments, misalignment of body weight, and the inertia of the moving segments. During jogging, the path of body's centre of gravity is sinusoidal, moving twice in the vertical direction, so there are two peaks for each stride. At the same time, when the centre of gravity loses height, it loses also horizontal speed, and the kinetic and potential energies are in phase, so large changes occur in the resultant of both forms of energy at each step. However, a significant amount of mechanical energy is conserved stored as potential elastic energy in the tissues. Another mechanism to save energy is its transferring between segments by two-joint muscles.

In jogging, the movements of the joints are larger in the sagittal (or anteroposterior) plane, even though the movements in the coronal and transverse planes facilitate the stability and progress in the sagittal plane, respectively. The movements are as follows:

1.  Sagittal plane: the axis of rotation is medial-lateral and the movements are of flexion-extension.

    1.a. In the ankle: *support phase* –dorsiflexion (10°), plantar flexion (45°); phase of non support –dorsiflexion (45°).

    1.b. In the knee: *support phase* –flexion (20°), extension (18°); *phase of non support* – flexion (90°), extension (90°).

    1.c. In the hip: *support phase* –extension (35°); *phase of non support* – flexion (40°), extension (10°) (Milliron & Cavanagh, 1990; Mann et al. 1986).

    1.d. The pelvis has a rocking motion, respect to the anterior-superior iliac spine: forward or down and back or up. In the stance phase there are up and down movements; and in the no-support phase, down, up, and down.

2.  Transverse plane: the lower limb segments rotate around a vertical axis, the direction of rotation is outward or inward and its development is the same in the components of the lower extremity: pelvis, thigh, and leg, but their magnitudes vary. The swing phase is characterized by the internal rotation of each segment; the more distal segments rotate faster and in a greater degree than the proximal ones. The average rotation of the pelvis is 5° and that of the tibia and femur 9°, summing up a total of 23°. In support phase the external rotation continues and then, halfway, its direction changes.

3.  Coronal or frontal plane: the axis of rotation is anterior-posterior and the movements are of ab-adduction. The displacements of the pelvis and lower extremity in the frontal plane are not large but are very important to maintain balance. In the knee and ankle the movements are ab-adduction and are limited by the characteristics of the joints and the presence of lateral ligaments. During jogging, the hip is adducted during the support phase until half of it. In the swing phase occurs continuous abduction of the supporting leg and at half of the way, it changes its direction to adduction.

4.  The movements of the ankle with the tibiofibular and subtalar joints produce the movement of supination-pronation.

## 1.2. Anatomy of the joints

From a biomechanical perspective, the factors that dictate the movement are our inherent structure and alignment, the joint range of motion, and the muscle strength available. The joint range is partly defined by the anatomical structure. In the following, the peculiarities of the joints of the legs and their angular displacements during locomotion are described (Testut 1971, Inman 1981, Perry 1992, Behnke 2001).

Each of the lower extremities is a system of articulated segments, with its own mechanical characteristics. The different joints involved are: (1) lumbosacral, (2) the two hips, (3) the two knees, (4) the two ankles, (5) the subtalar joints, and (6) the midtarsal joints. In studies on locomotion the foot is considered as a rigid segment (although it is formed by 26 bones) serving for the transmission of force between the body and the ground. During the movement, the body segments serve as levers (Perry 1992).

According to Arsenault et al. (1987) it seems clear that the kinematics of locomotion does not show high variability. From the data found in the literature, we describe the angular movements of different segments: pelvis, thigh, leg, and foot of the lower extremity in three planes: sagittal, coronal, and transverse during the different phases of the cycle locomotion.

In the sagittal plane, the movements are wider. In the other two planes the movements are small but are involved in the magnitude of the displacement of the center of gravity in the sagittal plane and also provide stability.

### 1.2.1. Ankle

The ankle is the only anatomical area where the vertical forces are transmitted to the horizontal support system, in this case the foot. The ankle includes the tibiofibular and the subtalar joints. The tibiofibular joint allows the movements of dorsiflexion and plantar flexion or extension in the sagittal plane. The lateral movement of the foot (or eversion) around the anterior-posterior and the medial movement (or inversion) are made in the subtalar joint in the frontal plane. Adduction and abduction movements occur around the vertical axis and the transverse plane. The combination of the movements of the tarsus with those of the ankle allows complex movements, such as: (1) supination, or inversion of the ankle with adduction of the foot and plantar flexion, and (2) pronation, or ankle eversion with abduction of the foot and dorsiflexion.

### 1.2.2. Knee

The knee is the binding site of two long bones, femur and tibia, which are the major body segments. Small range of motion produces significant changes in the foot or in the body.

The knee joint is very complex, bicondylar, characterized by a very wide range of motion in the sagittal plane and small arcs of motion in the coronal and transverse planes. During the movement of the knee in the sagittal plane, the tibia slides around the distal end of the femur so that the mediolateral axis of rotation displaces with movement.

The patella is the largest sesamoid bone in the human body. It modifies the thrust angle of the quadriceps femoris, affecting the production of muscle force components, so that the rotational component is greater (Nordin & Frankel, 2004).

During support, the knee is essential for the stability of the leg. During swinging, the flexibility of the knee is the main factor that determines the progress of the leg. The number of bicondylar muscles involved in controlling the knee indicates a great functional coordination with the hip and ankle.

The movement in the sagittal plane is used for progression through the support and during swing. During the phase of non support, the knee makes use of a range of movement widest than that of the any other joint. The rotation in the transverse plane accommodates changes in alignment when the body oscillates back and forth of the supporting leg. In walking, when the knee extends, the leg rotates externally; when the knee is flexed, the leg rotates internally. In jogging, the knee is flexed at the beginning of the stance phase while the leg is externally rotated (Novacheck 1998).

The movement in the coronal plane facilitates vertical balance on the leg, particularly during leg stance. In each cycle the knee moves into abduction and adduction. In support phase, the movement is of abduction. During oscillation, the knee returns to a more neutral position in adduction. In the transverse plane of a position of maximum external rotation at the end of the stance phase, the lower limb starts an internal rotation in the take-off of the leg and continues during the oscillation and the load response (initial part of the support phase).

### 1.2.3. Hip

The hip function differs from the other two joints in the following respects: (1) represents the junction between the passenger and the motor system, (2) allows movements in three planes of space with a specific control in each plane, although in the coronal plane movement is limited, but the mechanical demands are substantial.

In the sagittal plane hip extends in the phase of support and flexes in the non-support one. The hip has small arcs of motion in adduction and in abduction. At the initial contact of the heel with the ground, the hip is in adduced position. At the beginning of the swing phase, the hip is in a relative abduction of 5°. In the transverse plane, the internal rotation peak occurs at the end of the loading phase and maximum external rotation occurs at the end of the pre-swing phase.

### 1.2.4. Pelvis

During the stride, the pelvis moves in three directions asynchronously. The point of support is the hip of the leg that is in support. All its ranges of motion are small: in the sagittal plane it is a rocking motion of 4°; in the frontal plane, 7°; and in the transverse plane, 10°.

## 1.3. Differences in locomotion due to shoes

De Wit et al. (2000) describe different angular displacements of the knee and ankle when subjects ran barefoot and when running shod. During running, the body reacts to the external environment which produces the ground reaction force (GRF) that occurs in response to the force action transmitted by the leg in contact with the ground. The GRF reflects the net effect of the muscle action and the accelerations of the segments while the foot is in contact with the ground (Martin & Morgan 1992). All segments contribute to the total acceleration of the body in proportion to the acceleration of its centre of gravity and its relative mass.

The three components of the GRF (vertical, anterior-posterior, and medial-lateral) change their size when using footwear (Nigg 1983). The GRF reflects the acceleration and deceleration of the centre of gravity. The gravity eases the contact of the foot with the ground.

### 1.3.1. Vertical component (GRFv)

During movement, the GRFv varies above and below the body weight due to the positive and negative accelerations undergone by the body. The difference between the vertical component and the body weight is due to acceleration of the body. The direction of displacement of centre of gravity and acceleration influences also the magnitude of the vertical component.

The vertical component is biphasic and has a first peak of early impact (at 20ms after the impact), representing between 140% and 160% (and up to 200%) of body weight (BW), in the runners who touch the ground first with the heel, and a second peak in the stance phase, which appears at 80 ms and can almost triple the body weight. The two peaks have different slopes, the first very fast and the second more gradual. Contact time is about 0.25 s. The first peak is associated with heel strike and indicates pronation. It is surprising that this peak is smaller in magnitude than the second peak that is associated with the propulsion.

### 1.3.2. Antero-posterior component (GRF a-p)

When the foot contacts the ground, it is pushed forward and suffers a reaction force that slows it down. At the time the body passes over the foot that is resting on the ground, the horizontal component is zero. When the body moves over the foot which is resting, the foot is pushed against the ground and the antero-posterior component becomes positive, facilitating the forward propulsion. Its magnitude represents 50% of the BW during jogging.

### 1.3.3. Medial-lateral component (GRF m-l)

The medial-lateral component is the smallest of all components. It has two polarities, the first in reaction to the force transmitted by the foot on the medial direction, and the second in reaction to the force transmitted by the foot in the lateral direction. The polarity of this component of one leg is opposite to the polarity of this component in the contralateral leg. Thus the sign of the lateral component of the right foot would be first positive and then negative, and for the left foot would be reversed. The variation in magnitude of the vertical, antero-posterior, and medial-lateral components means that during the displacement, the speed is not constant, as the body moves faster in one point and slower in another.

The parameters related to the vertical component are the peak impact and the rate of increase of force (obtained with a force plate), and were used to examine the load under which the locomotor system is during locomotion (Nigg 1983). One of the main functions of the footwear is to cushion the strength of the action the subject exerts on the ground and to absorb the reaction force in order to protect the musculoskeletal system. In jogging, running shoes nullifies the impact peak and is involved in delaying the onset of the support vertical force by changing the gradient loading (Nigg 1983, De Wit et al. 2000). The anteroposterior force, which has two phases (braking and propulsion), is influenced by the friction introduced by the shoe sole. The medial-lateral component that guides us on the prono-supination movement can be modified by the shoes as they change the distance between the point of application of the GRF and the subtalar or calcaneo-talar joint.

Wakeling et al. (2001) speculated that the muscle activation levels in the lower extremities are adjusted depending on the loading speed of impact forces. Nigg & Wakeling (2001) suggested that the repetitive impact forces during physical activities are not responsible for possible injury but are the cause of changes in myoelectric activity (activation time and amplitude), and these changes are responsible for the injury. Gollhofer & Komi (1987) found differences in the electrical activity of muscles when subjects ran barefoot first, then shod; Gavilanes & Goiriena-de-Gandarias (2004) found changes in myoelectric activity throughout the gait cycle when the subjects walked barefoot or with two different types of footwear, with no differences due to types of footwear used. Wakeling et al. (2002) found that the muscle activity concomitant to the impact can be altered by changing the hardness of the shoe. Frederick (1986) concluded that footwear induces adjustments in the movement of the legs, which in turn have secondary effects on the kinetics.

As found in the literature, footwear induces adaptations in the motion of the joints of the lower extremities, changes in the reaction force, and modifications in the myoelectric activity. When designing and making shoes, different types of considerations are taken into account: (1) reduce excessive burden, by absorbing the impact, (2) improve the dynamic stability, (3) increase the performance, and (4) feel comfortable (Ramiro et al. 1988, Segesser & Nigg 1993). The impact absorption is carried out through the midsole of sport shoes that acts as a filter by changing the impact forces (Luethi & Stacoff 1987). The increase in performance with the use of the shoe has been an argument used by athletes and shoe manufacturers. The midsole of athletic shoes is a layer of resilient, deformable material that is interposed between the upper shoe and the outside. The main function is to provide a protective layer between the foot and the ground and soften the shock of impact. During the first stage of the stride of jogging, the midsole is compressed by the pressure of the foot and the forces acting on it do some work on the viscoelastic material of the sole. Part of this work becomes stored as deformation energy in the material (elastically deformed). When the load on the midsole is reduced, the material undergoes an elastic recovery to its original shape (Shorteen 1993).

The literature review reveals as well that the ability of sport shoes to mitigate the impact forces between the ground and the body has been examined by different researchers (Denoth et al. 1981, Bates et al. 1983, Nigg et al. 1986, Gollhofer & Komi 1987, Dufek JS et al. 1991, Forner et al. 1995, De Wit et al. 2000). Less studied are the effects of footwear on kinematics (Frederick 1986, Nigg et al. 1986), or muscle activity (Gollhofer & Komi 1987, Wakeling et al. 2001, Nigg & Wakeling 2001, Wakeling et al. 2002, Gavilanes & Goiriena de Gandarias 2004).

The design of sport shoes and the elasticity of the materials used in their sole influence, respectively, the location of the application point of the GRF and its magnitude. These parameters influence the ability to produce an angular movement of the joints. The elasticity of the materials can be characterized based on the concepts of elasticity, rigidity, deformability, hysteresis, resilience, and viscosity. Elasticity: ability of a body to recover its original shape once the force that has deformed it has disappeared. Stiffness: a body resistance to deformation. Deformability: the inverse of the stiffness, requiring little force per unit area to produce large deformation. Hysteresis: represents the energy dissipated between the deformation and recovery of the original shape. Resilience: the amount of energy returned by the deformed material during the discharge phase. Viscosity of a liquid or semiliquid substance is the resistance of a body to deformation in response to a load.

The duration of each phase of the jogging stride (support, flight, and swing) depends on the control of the muscles of each leg executed by the Nervous System: suprasegmental centres, spinal networks, and afferent information from the different senses and from the osteoarticular system. If the information from the feet changes due to modifications on the interface between the foot and the floor, it is expected that the muscular activity will be also modified.

The recording of electrical activity obtained during muscle contraction or electromyogram (EMG) reflects the muscle involvement in the movement of the joints and therefore in the kinetic response of the ground or reaction force. The EMG amplitudes are related both to the nervous system and to muscle tension, although the response of the mechanical system is not directly related to the nervous system signal (Bouisset 1973), as the mechanical response depends on more variables than the muscle activity (such as the length of the muscle, the rate of change of length, time of contraction, and the lever arm magnitude). The relationship between muscle activity and force is not straightforward; however, EMG amplitude, duration, and coordination among different muscles can provide information about the neural and mechanical systems. Therefore, the electromyography is a powerful tool in the study of the neuromusuclar control of movement. The EMG signal is not easily recorded, as it is very susceptible to interferences and cable movement, and it is quite small, varying its amplitude between microvolts and millivolts (Kleissen et al. 1998) being its maximum amplitude (peak-to-peak) only 5 mV when using surface electrodes (Winter 1979).

During locomotion, the muscles of the legs are used to meet the following mechanical demands: progression, dynamic stability, and improving the impact and energy conservation (Inman et al. 1981); if any of these tasks is altered, the record of the muscles electrical activity will provide information about its contribution.

The aim of our present study was to evaluate the influence of footwear on the electrical activity of muscles of both legs when running barefoot and running with two different types of sports footwear, in order to assess the effects on: the extent of muscle electrical signal, the profile of muscular electrical activity, the order of muscle involvement, and the coactivation of antagonist muscles.

## 2. Material and methods

### 2.1. Subjects

Ten (six male and four female) healthy subjects, 19 and 20 years old, with an average height of 1.73±0.10 m, with no history of neurological or musculoskeletal dysfunction, voluntarily participated in the study. All of them gave their written informed consent before participating in this research.

## 2.2. Experimental conditions

We have classified the hardness of the sole of each footwear type during jogging on the basis of their subjective hardness: barefoot condition was interpreted as the maximum hardness, as the outer protection and reduction of the shock at the beginning of the stance phase was minimal. The own athletic shoes of each subject (typically used to run) was the condition interpreted as the softest. The standard shoes were harder than the athletic shoes, and therefore feature less cushioning of the impact.

## 2.3. Proceeding

Prior to obtaining EMG recordings, subjects got used to carrying the electrodes and contact sensors (foot switches –FS) by walking freely in the laboratory until obtaining a normal gait.

For each individual there have been five successive records barefoot at spontaneous speed (no specific speed requested), five with a standard sports shoes and five with his/her own shoes. Subjects ran at ground level at their preferred speed in both the first registration and in the remaining four. When subjects were shod, they were given also some time to get habituated to the shoes, and moved at a freely chosen speed.

Each record registered the EMG corresponding to the cycles required to cross a distance of 10 m. From the cycles registered, clearly identified by the FS signal, only the central 2 were further analyzed; thus avoiding the effect of acceleration and deceleration on muscle activity. In order to calculate the average speed (in $ms^{-1}$), the time taken to cross the 10 m has been timed. Between each of the five records made for each condition, a pause of one minute was given.

The eight FSs (B & L, U.S.A.) facilitated the identification of the phases of the stride for each of the lower extremities. These sensors are flexible disks of two sizes: 18mm and 30mm. They were placed under the heel (30mm FS) and on the heads of the first and fifth metatarsal and toe tip (18mm FS). When subjects were shod, the FSs were placed on the bottom of the shoes at the sites corresponding to the outer edge of the heel, first and fifth metatarsal, and toe tip. A FS is activated when a pressure greater than 150 g is applied on it.

## 2.4. EMG

Visual monitoring of the signal from the FS eased the removal of stride records with deficiencies. The simultaneous recording of signals originating in the FS and the EMG has also allowed identifying the cycle phases (support, swing, or flight) in which the muscles were active. Prior to the start of the records, we checked the signals obtained through the electrodes and the FSs.

The electrode characteristics are presented in **Table 1**. The surface electrodes used were active, equipped with pre-amplifiers providing a gain of x320. EMG signal thus obtained is better than that achieved with passive electrodes respect to the level of noise. They are composed of three stainless steel electrodes, acting two as active electrodes and one as a common ground.

The leads used were bipolar, recording the difference signal between the two active electrodes ends. A general reference electrode was located on the right forearm of each subject.

| Body size | 50mm x 18mm x 7mm |
|---|---|
| Inter-electrode distance | Three 1/2" (1.27 cm) disks on 11/16" (0.16 cm) centres |
| Weight | 30 grams (including connector) |
| Connector | LEMO, 5 pin male style |
| Cable Length | 60 inches (1.5 metres) |
| Input Impedance | Greater than 100 MΩ |
| CMRR | >100dB at 60Hz |
| Bandwidth | 10 Hz to 30KHz (-3dB) |
| Gain at 1kHz | 320 |
| Power Requirements | ±4V to ±14V at 200μA |

**Table 1.** Technical specifications of the active, surface electrodes used in this study.

The electrodes chosen for the study were of surface type, because they have the following advantages over intramuscular ones: do not cause pain or bleeding, are easier to apply, and as shown by Kadaba et al. (1985), they provide a more reproducible signal than that obtained with intramuscular electrodes.

The subject carried on his back a box with 14 channels (12 for EMG signal input from the 12 target muscles) and 2 for the signal from the FSs. Each channel had an additional gain range of 1 to 8. The 14 signals were transmitted through a optic fibre cable from the junction box to the electromyograph, a Motion Lab MA200 system equipped with a Pentium PC 64 MB of RAM, a CODAS acquisition card PGH DI 400, with 16 channel and 12 bit resolution. Through the Motion Lab software 900, reports of the actual electrical activity have been obtained and the linear envelop (LE) has been calculated. Afterwards, each LE has been expressed with respect to the normalized gait cycle. The display of the EMG signal in real time while being recorded has allowed us to assess the quality of the recording during movement, ensuring a good contact between the electrode and the skin and the absence of artefacts. The acquisition system (200 Motion Lab) has the following characteristics: level of signal output ± 5 V, bandwidth of 20 Hz to 1000 Hz, CMMR of 40 dB, and input impedance of 100 Ω.

The 12 muscles whose activity has been recorded have been forcibly superficial, as we were using surface electrodes. Four muscles were proximal: rectus femoris (RF), vastus medialis (VM), biceps femoris (BF) long portion, semitendinosus (ST); and two distal: tibialis anterior (TA) and lateral gastrocnemius (GN, or calf). These muscles were selected for their synergistic action and agonist-antagonist relationships. Biarticular muscles: rectus femoris, long head of biceps femoris, semitendinosus, and gastrocnemius; monoarticular: vastus medialis; through one of the joints examined: tibialis anterior. Architectural features of the muscles under study are shown in **Table 2**, and their function and innervation are shown in **Table 3**.

| Muscle | Mass (g) | Muscular Length (ML) [mm] | Fibre Length (FL) [mm] | Pennation Angle [º] | Cross section area [cm2] | FL/ML |
|---|---|---|---|---|---|---|
| Rectus Femoris | 84,3±14 | 316±5.7 | 66.0±1.5 | 5.0±0.0 | 12.7±1.9 | 0.209±0.002 |
| Vastus Medialis | 175±41 | 335±15 | 70.3±3.3 | 5.0±0.0 | 21.1±4.3 | 0.210±0.005 |
| Tibialis Ant. | 65,7±10 | 298±12 | 77.3±7.8 | 5.0±0.1 | 9.9±1.5 | 0.258±0.015 |
| Biceps Femoris | 128±28 | 342±14 | 85.3±5 | 0.0±0.0 | 12.8±2.8 | 0.251±0.022 |
| Semitendinosus | 76.9±7.7 | 317±4 | 158±2 | 5.0±0.0 | 5.4±1.0 | 0.498±0.0 |
| Gastrocnemius | 150±14 | 248±9.9 | 35.3±2 | 16.7±4.4 | 32.4±3.1 | 0.143±0.010 |

**Table 2.** Architectural characteristics of the studied muscles (from Wickiewiz et al. 1983).

The location of the electrodes was done by orienting the surfaces of the electrodes with respect to the direction of muscle fibres (Testut 1971, Wickiewiz et al. 1983, Lieber 1992), in order to obtain a signal of greater amplitude and frequency (De Luca 1997). The electrodes were placed following the recommendations of SENIAM (1999). Electrodes location was verified by performing specific muscular contractions before carrying out the records.

| Muscles | Joint | Function (at each Plane) | | | Innervation |
|---|---|---|---|---|---|
| | | Sagittal | Coronal | Transversal | |
| Rectus Femoris | hip | flexor | abductor | | Crural Nerve L2-L4 |
| | knee | extensor | | | Crural Nerve L2-L4 |
| Vastus Medialis | knee | extensor | | | |
| Biceps Femoris | hip | extensor | adductor | external rotator | Sciatic Nerve L4-S2 |
| | knee | flexor | | external rotator | |
| Semitendinosus | hip | extensor | adductor | internal rotator | Sciatic Nerve L4-S2 |
| | knee | flexor | | internal rotator | |
| Tibialis Anterior | tibiofibular-talar | flexor | | | Tibial Nerve L4-S1 |
| | subtalar | | inverter | adductor | |
| Gastrocnemius | knee | flexor | | | Tibial Nerve L4-S3 |
| | ankle | extensor | | | |

**Table 3.** Muscles targeted in this study: function and innervation (Kendall 2000).

The optimum recording of action potentials require excellent preparation of the skin before placing on it the electrodes; i.e., waxing the area, removing debris with alcohol, and letting it to air dry. Each electrode was attached to the skin via hypoallergenic tape and bandage.

## 2.5. Signals analysis

The EMG signals and those from the pressure sensors were recorded digitally at a frequency of 3000 samples per second using an analog-to-digital card CODAS (DataQ Instruments, OH, USA). The records were afterwards selected for further processing based on the signal obtained with the pressure sensors.

In order to determine the intensity of the signal, peak amplitude (peak activity), and time of its appearance, it is necessary to use quantitative methods on the EMG signal such as the LE. The steps to obtain it are: (1) complete (full-wave) rectification of the raw EMG, and (2) obtaining the linear envelop window (LE window) by calculating the average amplitude values contained in a moving window of 50 points.

Further processing was carried out with the signals of six subjects (the records of four subjects were excluded because their signals were not fully valid). From each record, the activity corresponding to 2 (out of 5) cycles were used (5x2 = 10), for 6 subjects (10 x 6 = 60), so 60 cycles were used in each condition. Since there are 3 different conditions, we analyzed a total of 180 (60 x 3) cycles. Therefore, the database consisted of 180 files; each file containing the 51 values of the LE corresponding to each of the 12 muscles and the time length of the phases of the cycle for both feet.

Each file has been then processes in a spreadsheet to obtain time-space parameters and the 51 values of each of the 12 muscles' EMG signals expressed in mV and corresponding to each 2% of the normalized length of jogging cycle.

For each subject, the LE corresponding to the 2% for each consecutive cycle locomotion were averaged across the 10 selected strides resulting in a pattern "ensemble average" of EMG (EAV), which represents an average pattern of the intra-subject LE. Using the EAV of all subjects, the Great Ensemble Average (GEAV) was obtained.

Muscle activity, represented by its LE, was expressed between the 0% and the 100% of the duration of the cycle. The maximum amplitude and time of peak onset were obtained from the GEAV.

## 2.6. Statistical analysis

The influence of footwear on speed, the phases of locomotion, right-left legs symmetry, general effort, and on the maximum amplitude of the EMG activity of the 12 target muscles was evaluated by analysis of variance (ANOVA) for one factor with the statistical package of Matlab (The MathWorks, Massachusetts, USA), using the following factorial model: footwear, with three levels (barefoot, shod with standard shoes, and shod with athletic shoes). The statistic F has been analyzed and the significance level considered was $p < 0.05$.

## 3. Results

The aim of our study was to evaluate the influence of footwear on the electrical activity of muscles of both legs when jogging barefoot and jogging with two types of footwear featuring different geometry and damping characteristics. The barefoot condition was interpreted as the one in which the external protection and shock reduction at the beginning of the stance phase were minimal. The standard shoe was harder than the athletic one, cushioning less the impact.

For the realization of this goal we propose more specific objectives: to determine the profile of the muscle electrical activity and the order of muscle participation, to detect changes in the amplitude of the electrical signal muscles, and to measure the level of coactivation of antagonistic muscles. The different phases of the gait cycle were measured based on the records obtained by the pressure sensors (see **Figure 1**) located under the foot or shoe sole.

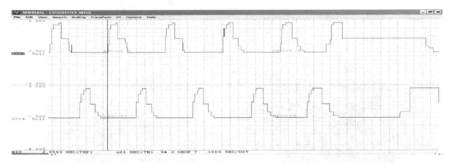

**Figure 1.** Bilateral support and non-support patterns from each foot obtained with pressure sensors.

The speed was higher when jogging with the own athletic shoes, and of a similar magnitude when jogging barefoot than when using standard sneakers. **Figure 2** shows the mean values of the speed and, for both legs, the mean values of the phases of: support, non support, and double flight. When running shod, the duration of the phases of the stride was different with respect the barefoot condition. The stance phase was shorter and the non-support phase, longer. The time length of the double flight increased. Between the two types of footwear used (standard and athletic) there were differences in speed but not in phases.

## 3.1. Muscular activity: EMG

**Figure 3** shows the EMG signal, processed and expressed as GEAV for the three conditions. To assess the influence of footwear, we have divided the stride into two phases: (1) support phase and (2) non-support phase, each of which exhibited its own characteristics in muscle activity.

In order to check whether there are differences in the muscular effort depending on the locomotion condition, we calculated the area under each muscle's GEAV for each condition and used it as an estimation of that effort. The ANOVA found that there is no statistically significant difference between the three conditions with respect to the general effort required for the locomotion.

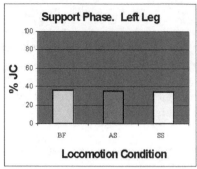

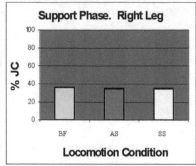

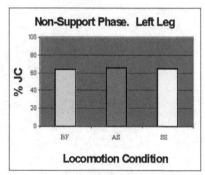

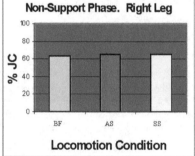

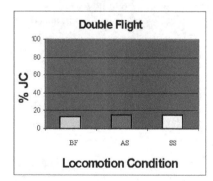

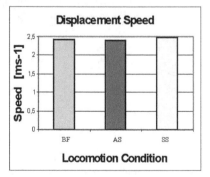

**Figure 2.** Space-temporal parameters expressed respect to the percentage of the jogging cycle (JC). Locomotion Conditions: BF –barefoot, AS –wearing athletic shoes, SS –wearing standard shoes.

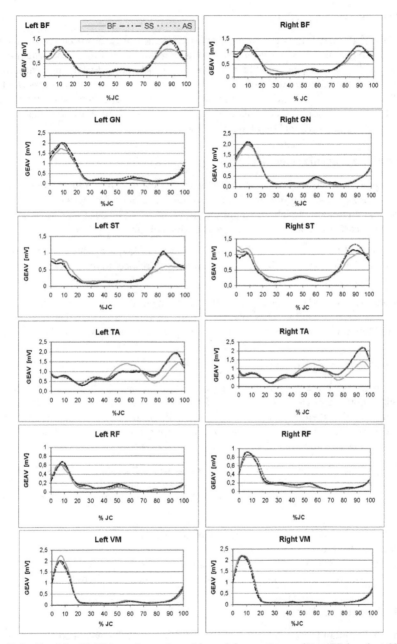

**Figure 3.** Profile of the GEAV for each muscle and for each locomotion condition (BF: barefoot, SS: standard shoes, and AS: athletic shoes).

## 3.2. Order of muscle participation

From the GEAV signal, the order of participation of each muscle can be seen. This order remained constant in all three conditions: tibialis anterior, hamstrings, gastrocnemius, and quadriceps. The AT muscle was the first one to be activated during the stride; it was activated before the flight of the ipsilateral foot, in the last part of unipodal support. The BF and ST were activated after the TA, but in the swing phase, i.e., when the contralateral leg was resting on the floor. The GN was activated in the final flight. Vastus medialis and RF were also activated in the final flight, but after the GN.

## 3.3. Profile of muscular electrical activity

The profile of the electrical activity is characterized by the length of time of muscle activity, the peak (maximum amplitude), and the time of its appearance. Changes in muscle activity can occur in any of the variables: amplitude, time, and frequency. In all three conditions muscle electrical activity was present for short periods of time.

The functions of the muscles varied through the cycle of jogging. There is no statistically significant difference between the three conditions with respect to the activity profile of the jogging cycle.

Rectus femoris, VM, and GN had a peak at the beginning of the stance phase. Tibialis anterior showed two peaks: one in the swing phase and another in the final flight. Biceps femoris and ST showed two peaks, one at the end of the non-support phase, and one in the initial support.

### 3.3.1. Time of onset of maximum intensity

**Table 4** gives the exact percentages of jogging cycle at which the maximum amplitude occurred. For five muscles there were no differences in the time of peak onset in their GEAV, maintaining their patterns of activity in the three conditions. As shown in Figure 3, the peak of the RF, VM, and GN appeared in the support phase; the peak of the BF, ST, TA, in the non-support phase.

In both legs, the peak appears in very similar times. Depending on the footwear, the time of occurrence of the peak is slightly modified. In general, muscles that have their peak after the impact when shod may appear a little later; and muscles that have their peak before impact when shod can occur earlier.

The peak of the RF, VM, and GN appeared between 6% and 10% in the three conditions and in both legs. The TA peaks between 94-96% in the final flight; the highest peak of the BF appeared between 88% and 90%. Semitendinosus peak appeared about 84%-90% in the shod condition, ahead respect to the barefoot condition, which appeared between 94-98%.

## 3.4. Maximum amplitude

The changes of amplitude or intensity of muscle activity can be evaluated considering: (1) the entire cycle, (2) the stance phase after impact, and (3) the non-support, before impact. We will describe the changes in that order.

| Locomotion condition | Left leg muscles | | | | | |
|---|---|---|---|---|---|---|
| | RF | VM | GN | TA | BF | ST |
| Barefoot | 8 | 6 | 8 | 96 | 90 | 98 |
| Standard shoes | 8 | 6 | 10 | 94 | 90 | 84 |
| Athletic shoes | 8 | 6 | 8 | 94 | 88 | 84 |
| Locomotion condition | Right leg muscles | | | | | |
| | RF | VM | GN | TA | BF | ST |
| Barefoot | 6 | 6 | 8 | 94 | 88 | 94 |
| Standard shoes | 6 | 8 | 10 | 94 | 90 | 88 |
| Athletic shoes | 10 | 6 | 10 | 94 | 90 | 90 |

**Table 4.** Time of occurrence (in % of the jogging cycle) of the GEAV peak in each of the three different locomotion conditions.

### 3.4.1. Maximum amplitude along the entire cycle

**Figure 4** shows the maximum activity displayed during the entire cycle by each of the twelve muscles. In all three conditions the muscles that had the highest amplitude were the VM, GN and TA. The muscles that showed less activity were the BF, ST and RF.

The maximum amplitude of homologous muscles was of the same order of magnitude for both legs, as shown in **Figure 5**.

There is no statistically significant difference between the three conditions with respect to the value of the amplitude peak.

### 3.4.2. Maximum amplitude during the support phase after impact

**Figure 6a** shows the maximum activity during the support phase produced after the impact of the heel. The TA, GN, and BF muscles in both legs increased their activity with both types of shoes. The behaviour of RF, VM, and ST varied positively and negatively.

The evolution of electrical activity in buffer muscles (RF and VM) during the loading phase was not the same in both legs, neither with both types of shoes.

**Figure 7** shows the increase (not normalized, in mV) of EMG activity with respect to the barefoot condition. When subjects wore standard shoes with hard soles, the RF of the left leg increased its maximum amplitude after impact, and the left VM decreased their activity.

When subjects wore their own shoes, the RF of the left leg decreased its peak amplitude after impact. The left VM decreased its activity; and the one of the right, increased.

When the shoe was harder, the left RF increased its activity and the VM of both legs decreased. When the shoe was softer, the RF of both legs and the VM of the left leg decreased its activity, and the right VM slightly increased its activity.

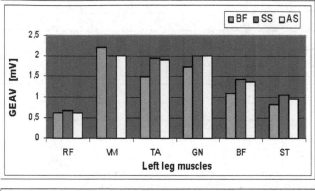

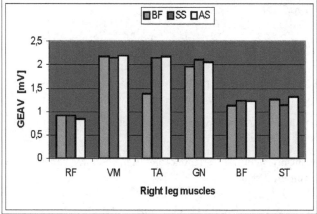

**Figure 4.** Peak of EMG during the whole cycle, for the left (upper graph) and right (bottom) legs muscles for each Locomotion Condition (BF: barefoot, SS: standard shoes, and AS: athletic shoes).

The TA of both legs increased their activity. The right TA increased more than the left one. In both legs, the TA increases more its maximum amplitude in the condition of own jogging shoes; perhaps because this type of shoe offers more cushioning. The GM activity in the condition of standard jogging shoe increased more than in the own shoe condition. When the hardness of the sole was higher, the translational velocity was lower and higher GM activity. Perhaps this trend has to do with balance, because when the speed is less, dynamic stability decreases.

The BF of both legs and both conditions increased their activity. In the standard shoe condition, it increased more. The ST in both conditions decreased its activity.

The response of the agonist muscles from the same muscle group is not the same when the shoe condition changes. Thus, with the standard shoe RF activity increased and decreased the one of VM, the BF increased, and ST decreased.

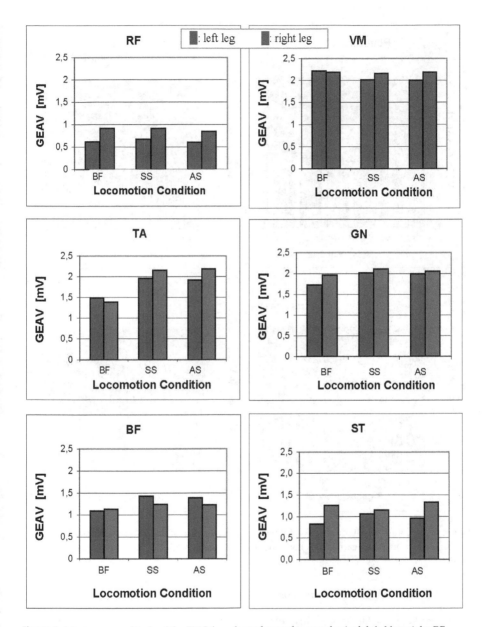

**Figure 5.** Maximum amplitude of the EMG from homologous leg muscles (red: left, blue: right; RF: rectus femoris, VM: vastus medialis, TA: tibialis anterior, GN: lateral gastrocnemius, BF: biceps femoris, ST: semitendinosus) for each locomotion condition (BF: barefoot, SS: standard shoes, and AS: athletic shoes).

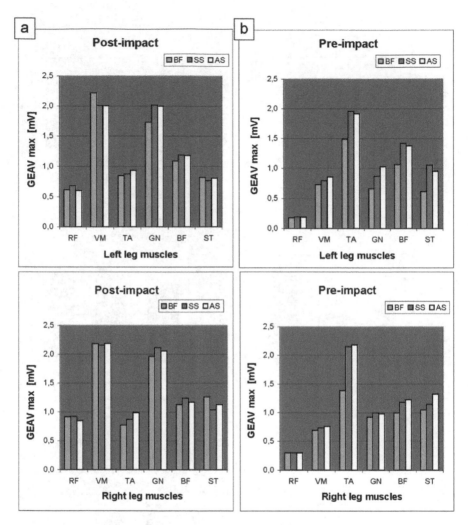

**Figure 6.** Maximum amplitude of the GEAV post - and pre-impact (after and before initial contact) for the 12 studied muscles for each locomotion condition (BF: barefoot, SS: standard shoes, and AS: athletic shoes).

### 3.4.3. *Maximum amplitude before impact*

As shown in **Figure 6b**, for both legs, five out of the six muscles (TA, GN, BF, ST, and VM) increased their activity in the non-support phase in shod condition. The RF maintained its level of activity; unlike what happened in the stance phase, in which the RF, VM, and ST decreased their activity.

**Figure 7** shows that the EMG signal before contact of the heel exhibited greater increase than in the signal after contact. The intensity of the myoelectric activity showed differences between both types of shoes. In both shod conditions the TA muscle activity increased more in absolute terms. The ST, BF and GN increased their activity more than the VM, the activity of which increased very little.

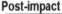

**Post-impact**

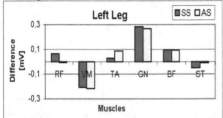 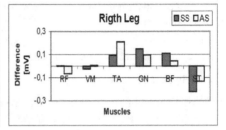

**Pre-impact**

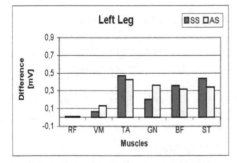 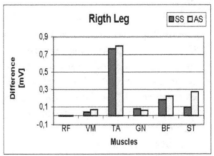

**Figure 7.** Absolute GEAV peaks amplitude increments respect to barefoot condition for the other two locomotion conditions (SS: standard shoes and AS: athletic shoes) for both legs muscles after impact (upper graph) and before impact (bottom graph).

In the left leg, the TA, BF, and ST were more active in the standard shoe condition. The increased activity of the semitendinosus was more important than that of the biceps femoris. In the right leg, the TA, BF, ST, and VM activity increased more in the athletic shoe condition than in the standard shoe condition. The electrical activity of the muscles of both legs showed different evolution depending on the type of shoe.

## 3.5. Activity of antagonist muscles

In order to evaluate the coactivity of agonist-antagonist muscles, we have established an index obtained as the ratio between the peak of the agonist muscle activity and the activity of the oppose muscle or muscles (antagonists). That index can be higher (agonist's peak is bigger than that of the antagonist) or below (opposite case) one (see **Figure 8**). To establish the role of a muscle as agonist or antagonist, we rely on the movement of joints:

- In the support phase, between 6% and 10% of the jogging cycle, the peaks of the following muscles occur: GN, RF, and VM; there is also a second peak of lesser magnitude in the activity of the BF and ST muscles. Concomitant to the important activity of these muscles, ankle dorsiflexion, knee flexion, and hip extension occur.
- In the phase of non support, the peak of the TA, BF, and ST are concomitant with an ankle dorsiflexion, knee extension, and hip extension.

There is no statistically significant difference between the three conditions with respect to the level of coactivation.

### 3.5.1. Coactivation during support phase

#### 3.5.1.1. Barefoot

- Coactivation of tibialis anterior (agonist) / gastrocnemius (antagonist): the peak activity of GN occurs between 8% and 10% of the jogging cycle. The TA shows no peak in the stance phase. The index is below unity. The LG shows greater activity during dorsiflexion.
- Coactivation of hamstring (agonist) / rectus femoris (antagonist): index above unity. The BF (hip extensor) shows increased activity.
- Coactivation of hamstring (agonist) BF / vastus medialis (antagonist): the index is less than unity and therefore smaller than that showed by the antagonist muscles BF and RF because the activity of VM is much higher.
- Coactivation of semitendinosus (agonist) / rectus femoris (antagonist): index greater than one, but less than that found between the BF and RF because the ST has less activity than the BF.
- Coactivation of semitendinosus (agonist) / vastus medialis (antagonist): the index is less than unity and therefore is less than that presented by the antagonist muscles BF and RF because the ST activity was smaller than that of the BF, and the activity of the VM is much higher.

The peaks of RF and VM were not taken into account because they occur while acting as antagonists.

#### 3.5.1.2. Shod

- Coactivation of tibialis anterior (agonist) / gastrocnemius (antagonist): both muscles increase their activity, so the index remained similar.
- Coactivation of semitendinosus (agonist) / vastus medialis (antagonist): the index is maintained because the two muscles decrease their respective activity.
- Coactivation of hamstring (agonist) / vastus medialis (antagonist): the index increases slightly because the BF activity increases and that of the VM decreases.
- Coactivation of semitendinosus (agonist) / rectus femoris (antagonist): the index decreases because the ST activity decreases.
- Coactivation of biceps femoris (agonist) / rectus femoris (antagonist): the index decreases because the RF activity increases.

The antagonist muscles showed more activity than agonist ones in the ankle and knee joints, for all the three conditions. In the hip, agonist muscles were more active, mainly in shod condition.

### 3.5.1.3. Coactivation during non-support phase

In the ankle and knee joints, agonist muscles showed a slightly higher activity than the antagonists. In the hip and knee, agonist muscles activity was higher.

The peaks of TA, BF, and ST muscles occur in the non-support phase (see Figure 3), concomitant with the dorsiflexion, the extension of the knee, and the hip extension. In all three conditions, the agonist muscles show greater activity than the antagonist muscles, as shown by the coactivity index being higher than one (see Figure 8). The results about the muscular coactivity during jogging barefoot and shod are just preliminary, but indicate that it is worth a study in greater depth on the subject.

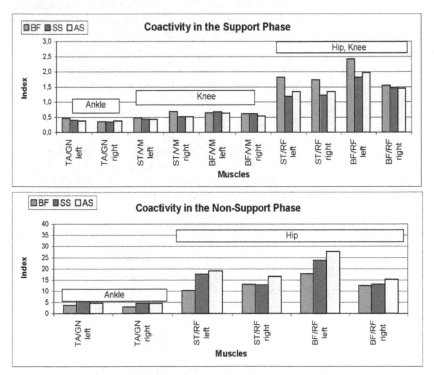

**Figure 8.** Coactivity of ago- and antagonist muscles during support (upper graph) and non-support (bottom graph) phases.

## 4. Discussion

The aim of our study was to evaluate the influence of footwear on the electrical activity of muscles of both legs when jogging barefoot and shod with two types of shoes, with different geometry and damping features. Our findings show that shoes increase the intensity of muscle activity, especially in the non-support phase. These results are consistent with those of Nigg et al. (2003) that showed specific changes in the intensity of muscle activation before heel strike.

The speed increase is concomitant with decreased activity of the VM and ST in the stance phase. The increase in the intensity of TA in the stance phase is less than in the non-support phase, a result consistent with Komi et al. (1987).

The speed of jogging at which the EMG activity was recorded in the three conditions was freely chosen by the subjects because previous research (e.g., Kadaba et al. 1985) have shown that EMG activity is more reproducible when the speed is chosen freely than when it is imposed.

We note that the footwear influences the speed of locomotion, increasing it in the athletic shoe condition. This result suggests that the speed has to be one more parameter to consider when assessing the influence of footwear on the interaction between man-shoe-surface. The speed in similar condition of hardness (barefoot and standard shoe) was similar, but muscle activity was different in both conditions, being more similar that of the standard shoe and athletic shoe conditions.

In the different conditions under study, the pattern of muscle activity kept its profile. The starting and ending times of the activity were constant, but the amplitude of the EMG signal changed when using footwear. Also, the duration of the phases in the shod condition was reversed with respect to the bare condition, decreasing the stance phase and increasing the non-support one.

A limitation of this work was that has considered only 6 muscles out of the 57 having each of the lower extremities. The advantage over previous studies is that it has analyzed those six muscles from both legs simultaneously. The fact that the homologous muscles of both legs have similar amplitude allows us to use their absolute values.

The timing of muscle activity was assessed using visual inspection of the actual records, which is the detection method used to interpret the real surface EMG signal. Usually, visual inspection provides a high level of accuracy because all the details of the signal can be measured. Detecting the beginning and end of the activity by using different types of algorithms is based on establishing a threshold, usually based on intuitive criteria. In the end, both visual interpretation and detection using algorithms are based on subjective criteria. The advantage of the subjectivity of the experimenter is based on the acquisition of the ability to interpret the EMG signal and experience that allows the evaluator to use the capabilities of the human brain to perform a more sophisticated interpretation of highly variable data (Staude & Wolf 1999).

The order of participation of the muscles studied did not vary with the type of shoes. First, the TA muscles activated, afterwards the muscles of the posterior part of the thigh (BF and ST), followed by the activation of the GN of the back of the leg, and finally the activation of the RF and VM of the anterior part of the thigh.

The length of time of muscle activity in the three conditions did not vary with respect to the normalized jogging cycle. In all conditions, muscle activity was present in the first half of the stance phase, disappearing in the second, when the body weight fell on the forefoot. In absolute values, the time of activity would be different because the stance phase was shorter in the condition of athletic shoes and the phase of non support was longer. Thus, the time of muscle activity would be greater in the stance phase and lower in the non-support phase.

It is interesting to find that during the jogging, as happens in walking, there are phases in which no muscle activity is taking place, although there are movements that would make one expect some muscular activity. This result is consistent with other studies that have shown that the main goal of locomotion is to transport the body from one position to another using lower limb locomotor coordination and effective mechanisms. The nervous system integrates the movement of different body segments and controls the activity of the muscles to decrease energy expenditure (Inman 1968).

This lack of muscle activity is not surprising. In jogging, the decrease of kinetic and potential energies in the first part of the support is concomitant with the accumulation of elastic energy in the tendons of the muscles; this energy is later released during the remainder of the stance phase to facilitate the progression and stability dynamics. Margaria and Cavagna (1965) found that during jogging, elasticity accounts for 50% of the work. During the unipodal support, the contralateral leg swing provides a second pushing force generated by the acceleration of the leg. Once the centre of gravity has shifted over the foot on the ground, the weight of the body becomes a driving force. When the contralateral leg is slowed by the hamstring muscles, the ipsilateral leg acquires kinetic energy, which is used to start the double flight. Inman (1968) argues that the slowdown of the swing leg during walking can contribute more to the forward movement of the body that the thrust of the ipsilateral leg. Once the leg is in motion, as the first law of Newton states, a force is needed to stop it, and that is the role of the hamstrings when they become active at the end of the swing phase. While the hamstrings are active, the RF and VM become activated to improve the accuracy of the landing of the foot.

The amplitude of the myoelectric activity, expressed in absolute values, varied when using the two different types of footwear; these results are consistent with those found by Gollhofer & Komi (1987), who found differences in the electrical activity of muscles when subjects were at first barefoot and then shod. The effects of athletic shoes on the amplitude of muscle activity were significant. Changes in hardness and shape of the shoe did not affect the muscle activity.

Different considerations have led us to not normalize the EMG signal amplitude: (1) to assess absolute muscle activity when a sole is interposed between the foot and the ground, and (2) to maintain the electrodes in place when the geometry of the footwear and the elasticity of the sole varied.

The subjects ran faster in the athletic shoe condition and muscle activity was similar in the two footwear conditions: higher in the non-support phase. There is no statistically significant difference between the three conditions with respect to the speed of locomotion.

There was similar muscle activity in both shod conditions, which was different from the barefoot condition. In this paper we have classified the hardness of footwear subjectively. Although the interaction subject-shoe-ground occurs only during the stance phase, the intensity of the EMG activity was modified both during the stance phase and during the phase of non support. At first, one might think that the presence of the sole alters the physical characteristics of the force of action and reaction and influences the feedback mechanisms of muscle activity. The results show that although the interaction subject-shoe-ground occurs only during the stance phase, the amplitude of the EMG activity was modified both in the stance and in the swing phases, the major changes occurring in the non-support phase.

Before the foot contacts the ground, there is no information available from the ground; therefore, no feedback mechanism is in use and muscle activity would be controlled by forward mechanisms. The changes in the amplitude of muscle activity in the two footwear conditions were more homogeneous in both legs during the post-impact than during the pre-impact. This finding is in agreement with those of Nigg (2003), who suggests that the EMG activity before and after impact corresponds to two different events. Before the foot contact with the ground, there is no information available from the ground, then no feedback mechanism is in use. It is speculated that this would be some pre-programmed muscle activity based on the expected impact and would be related to the "muscle tuning" and controlled by a forward mechanism. Thus, the configuration of the leg when the heel hits the floor is prepared beforehand during the non-support phase, following the strategy adopted (De Wit et al. 2000). In the other hand, the activity that appears after heel contact is due to a reflex effect. In this context, one can understand the variability of electrical activity in the pre-impact and its consistency in the post-impact.

The changes in the impact force described under the influence of footwear may be a consequence of changes in muscle activity in the non-support phase to reduce soft tissue vibrations during locomotion. Wakeling et al. (2002) explains how the frequencies of the impact force and the soft tissues may overlap during walking and running. It can be expected that the impact forces will cause vibrations within the range of vibration of the soft tissues. However, observations show that such vibrations are minimal. Wakeling et al. (2002) proposed that muscle activity is adjusted before impact in order to reduce possible vibrations resulting from the impact.

The reflex effect has to be understood in the context that the heel contact with the ground is a stimulus that triggers feedback mechanisms. This stimulus does not trigger the onset of muscle activity, which had already begun in all muscles during the swing phase or during the final flight phase (or even during the initial flight phase), but could just change it. The reflex time is around 110 ms in the normal population (Kroll & Clarson 1978), and is divided into a latency time of 20 ms and a motor time of 90 ms. A peak muscle activity for most of the muscles studied appears on the 8% of 700ms-long jogging cycle, i.e. at 56 ms, which correspond well with the reflex motor time.

The maximum activity peak appears in the three conditions in the same phase. The increase in mean activity increased recruitment of motor units and increased force production. The decrease means the opposite. The observation of decreased activity of the VM in the post-impact is consistent with previous findings (De Wit et al. 2000) about the influence of shoes on the ground reaction force. In the shod condition, impact peak appears later perhaps due to decreased activity of the damper (shock absorber) muscles. The loading speed is influenced by muscle activity, which affects the acceleration of the segments.

When wearing footwear, the right and left BF increased their activity at the end of the swing phase, in the final flight, and in the onset of the stance phase. At the end of the swing phase, those muscles act as antagonists of the extension of the knee and of the hip flexion in the swing phase; from the final flight phase, they act as agonists of the extension of the hip.

The increased activity of BF in the shod condition at the end of the swing phase could be justified by the higher speed and greater participation of these muscles to slow down the flexion of the thigh. In principle, its action would facilitate the advancement of the leg by inertia, and then its action would stop the leg being extended to facilitate the support of the foot on the floor. Perhaps, the increased activity in the phase of non-support has an effect on increasing the speed of the contralateral leg, as suggested by the studies of Inman (1968). At the beginning of the stance phase, the BF and ST intervene as agonists of the extension of the hip and knee flexion, cooperating synergistically with the torque that has the lower extremity and maintained as a result of inertia when the foot has been slowed by friction with the ground. When the sole absorbs more impact, shock muscles (RF and VM) decreased its activity. When the shoe was harder, the left RF increased its activity and that of the VM of both legs decreased.

The fact that the muscles of both legs do not modify its maximum amplitude in the same percentage is understood in the context that the activity of a leg is adapted to the activity of the other. However, in the left leg there are significant differences in the activity of some of its muscles when wearing different types of footwear (see for example O'Connor 2005).

The lower activity of the RF and of the VM observed at the beginning of the stance phase may facilitate hip extension and knee flexion caused by increased activity of the hamstrings. This finding is consistent with the results of De Wit et al. (2000) who found that the knee is more flexed in the medium supporting phase in the shod condition. Also in that condition, the TA increased its activity in the final flight and at the beginning of the stance phase, being its activity lower during part of the swing. The role of the TA in the final flight and at the beginning of the stance phase is to promote dorsiflexion. The increased activity in the final flight can be explained based on segmental geometry: the hip extends and the foot flexes dorsally to avoid bumping into the ground until the proper stride length has been obtained. When jogging without shoes, De Wit et al. (2000) reported increased plantar flexion at the beginning of the support phase. Our results are consistent with their findings: the lower activity of the TA muscle in this condition would favour plantar flexion, apparently intended to reduce the pressure, which is higher in the barefoot condition because the impact force is increased and occurs in a shorter time.

One explanation for the decreased activity of ST in the stance phase in the shod condition could be the following: this muscle is extensor and adductor of the hip, and also flexor and rotator of the knee. Shod, the movement from supine-pronation can be affected by the change in the distance between the point of application of the GRF and the subtalar or calcaneus-talus joint. The shoes would favour a faster decrease of the inversion with a faster rotation of the knee in a lower limb that is externally rotated, favouring a twist in the knee. If the ST does not decrease its activity, it would increase that twisting torque affecting the knee. A more active GN in the stance phase could influence the stability of the ankle. In the shod condition, there is more damping of the impact force. Cushioning and stability are conflicting (Perry 1992): more cushioning brings less stability.

Nigg et al. (2003) speculated that the body reacts to changes in input signal to adapt the muscle activity to reduce the vibrations of the soft tissues. In principle, the proximal muscles would be less required than the distal ones. These authors found that the TA activity increased more than that of the proximal ones (BF and ST). Our results are consistent with those findings respect to the TA and the ST; but not for the BF.

According to Mundermann et al. (2003), changes in the intensity of leg muscles activity predict better the differences in comfort than changes in the impact force. As the muscle activity decreased in the stance phase, the kinematic differences between the conditions disappeared (De Wit et al. 2000). This result is consistent with the absence of muscle activity. The signal amplitude indicates the level of activation of the muscle: there is a relationship between activity and strength, implying that increased activity is the source of increased muscle strength. The change in muscle electrical activity may be due to the role of the muscles to adapt to the characteristics of elasticity and friction of the shoes used.

According to Arsenault et al. (1987), it seems clear that the kinematics of locomotion is not very variable. From the scientific literature one can obtain the parameters describing the movement and explain muscle activity during jogging in different conditions. When the peak of the RF, VM, GN, BF, and ST muscles appears, the hip stretches, the knee flexes, and the ankle flexes dorsally. Rectus femoris and VM undergo an eccentric contraction, BF and ST concentric, and GN concentric in the knee and eccentric in the ankle. Biceps femoris and GN promote the flexing of the knee and the GN transfers energy from the ankle to the knee.

The activation of the muscles acting as antagonists (i.e., contracting eccentrically) promote the absorption of energy recovered in the immediate concentric contraction. In the condition barefoot, the BF presented electrical activity at the end of the swing phase, in the final flight, and at the onset of stance phase, acting first as antagonist and then as agonist. With shoes, the activity increased in both phases, increasing the energy absorbed in the non-support phase. During the concentric contraction at the beginning of the stance phase, the increased activity means more power generation. The increase of the absorbed energy and the energy produced could be interpreted as an effort at the beginning of the stance phase in order to do hip extension, perhaps to counterbalance the increased frictional force that opposes the advance in the shod condition. At the beginning of the support phase, the GN, RF, and VM are active in eccentric contraction. The reduction of the duration of the support phase in the shod condition may improve the efficacy of the stretching-shortening cycle.

The potential problem of crosstalk was reduced using a double differential technique, which is based on a single amplifier fed with three electrodes (De Luca & Merletti, 1988; Winter, 1990; Winter et al., 1994). It is already widely accepted that double-differential technique reduces the level of cross-talk (see, *e.g.*, De Luca & Merletti, 1988; and Meinecke et al., 2004). In any case, cross-talk cannot ever be fully cancelled.

As the human body is a biological system that has many possibilities of action and reaction, it would be advisable to evaluate the electrical activity of other additional muscles when changing the subject-shoe-ground interface. According to Ferris et al. (1999), persons adjust the degree of stiffness of the legs when they run on different surfaces. The stiffness is given by the coactivation of the ago-antagonists muscles that cross the joints. In the support phase, the coactivation in the shod condition was greater than in the barefoot condition. At the stage of non support, the coactivation in the shod condition was not homogeneous, neither for both legs nor for all muscles, as it may decrease or increase respect to the barefoot condition.

A major function of footwear is to cushion both the strength of action the subject performs on the ground and absorb its reaction force, in order to protect the musculoskeletal system. Athletic shoes diminish –or even nullify- the impact peak of the vertical component and are involved in delaying the onset of the vertical support force, by changing the load gradient (Nigg 1983, De Wit et al. 2000).

The impact force acts as an input signal in the body and influences the vibration of the soft tissues (Nigg et al. 2000). The vertical component is biphasic and has two peaks: the impact peak appears after 20 ms of the impact, representing 140-160% -200% of BW, in those runners that support the heel first in the ground. A second peak, in the stance phase, appears at 80 ms and can almost triple the BW. Previous works (De Wit et al. 2000, Nigg 1983) have shown that in jogging, the magnitude of the passive and active peaks of the vertical component of the GRF does not vary with the shoes. The load gradient was lower in the shod condition due to the later occurrence of the impact force (33 ms against 11 ms).

In our study, peak muscle activity appeared in the following cycle time: 2-6% for the ST, 6-8% for the VM and RF, 8-10% for GN. In absolute values, the 2% amounts to 14 ms, 6% to 42 ms, and 10% to 70 ms. The activity peak of four muscles occur between the peaks of the vertical component of the reaction force. Despite finding a second peak of greater magnitude in the shod condition, muscle activity was higher in only three of the six muscles studied. In two of the other muscles (VM and ST) in the shod condition the activity was lower. In the RF, the activity response was not constant.

The increased activity of the TA in the shod condition could lead to the appearance of the anterior compartment syndrome of the lower leg. The results here presented about the increased EMG signal amplitude suggest further studies to corroborate or refute the argument used by athletes and shoe manufacturers on increased performance with the use of athletic footwear.

## Author details

Begoña Gavilanes-Miranda
*Faculty of Physical Activity and Sport Science, University of Basque Country, Vitoria, Spain*

Juan J. Goiriena De Gandarias
*Faculty of Medicine, University of Basque Country, Bilbao, Spain*

Gonzalo A. Garcia*
*Biorobotics Department, TECNALIA, Bilbao, Spain*

---

* Corresponding Author

## Acknowledgement

Authors thank the volunteers who participated in the experiments carried out for the present work. Thanks also to J. de la Cruz (Department of Applied Economy, University of Basque Country, Spain), F. Ainz (Department of Physiology, University of Basque Country, Spain), and to J. Bilbao (Department of Statistics, University of Basque Country, Spain) for their participation in the analysis of the data; and to S. Rainieri (Food Research Division, AZTI-Tecnalia, Spain) for helpful comments on the original manuscript.

This study was supported by the Foundation *Jesús de Gangoiti Barrera*. G.A.G. was supported by a European Marie Curie Post-doctoral Fellowship (ADCOMP project; Contract MEIF-CT-2006-025056). The CONSOLIDER INGENIO 2010 must be acknowledged for supporting partially this work through grant CSD2009-00067.

## 5. References

Arsenault AB, Winter DA, Marteniuk RG (1987). Is there a 'normal ' profile of EMG activity in gait?. Medical & Biological Engineering & Computing 337-343.

Bates BT, Osterninig JA, Sawhill JA (1983). An assessment of subject variability, subject inter-action, and the evaluation of running shoes using ground reaction force data. J Biomec 16: 181-191.

Behnke R (2001). Kinetic Anatomy. Human Kinetics, Champaign,IL.

Bouisset S (1973). EMG and force in normal motor activities. In: Desmedt JE ed. New developments in electromyography and clinical neurology. Base: Karger: 547-583.

De Luca CJ (1997). The use of surface electromyography in biomechanics. Journal of Applied Biomechanics 13: 135-167.

De Luca CJ & Merletti R. (1988). Surface myoelectric signal cross-talk among muscles of the leg. Electromyography and Clinical Neurophysiology; 1988, 69:568-75.

De Wit B, De Clercq D, Aerts P (2000). Biomechanical analysis of the stance phase during barefoot and shod running. J Biomech Mar;33(3):269-78.

Dufek JS, Bates BT, Davis HP, Malone LA (1991). Dynamic performance assessment of selected sport shoes on impact forces. Medicine and Science in Sports and Exercise 23 (9): 1062-1067.

Denoth J and Nigg B (1981). The influence of various sport floors on the load on the lower extremities. In : Biomechanics VII-B,A. Morecki, K Fidelus ,K Kedzior and A Wit (eds). Baltimore: University Park Press, 100-106.

Ferris DP, Liang K, Farley CT (1999). Runners adjust leg stiffness for their first step on a new running surface. J Biomech. 32: 787-794.

Forner A, Garcia AC, Alcantara E, Ramiro J, Hoyos JV, Vera P (1995). Properties of shoe insert materials related to shock wave transmission during gait. Foot Ankle Int Dec;16(12):778-86

Frederick EC (1986). Kinematically mediated effects of sport shoe design: a review. J Sports Sci 4 (3): 169-184.

Gavilanes MB, Goiriena de Gandarias JJ (2004). Muscle activity in shod and barefoot healthy young subjects during walking. In : International proceedings of XVth Congress of the International Society of Electrophysiology & Kinesiology. Boston U.S.A. 2004:105

Gollhofer A, Komi PV (1987). Measurement of Man-Shoe-Surface interaction during locomotion. Medicine Sport Sci, 26: 187-199.

Inman VT (1968). Conservation of energy in ambulation. In: Bull Procc Res BPR 1968; 10:(9):26-35.

Inman VT, Ralston HJ, Todd F (1981). Human walking. Baltimore, MD, Williams and Wilkins Company.

Kadaba MP, Wootten ME, Gainey J, Cochran GV (1985). Repeatability of phasic muscle activity: performance of surface and intramuscular wire electrodes in gait analysis. J Orthop Res. 1985;3(3):350-9.

Kendall FP, Mccreary EK, Provance PG (2000). Músculos: pruebas funcionales, postura y dolor. Willinams & Wilkins. Baltimore.

Kleissen RFM, Buurke JH, Harlaar J, Hof AL, Zilvold G. C (1998). Electromyography in the biomechanical analysis of human movement and its clinical application. Gait & Posture 8 : 143-158.

Komi PV, Gollhofer A, Schmidtbleicher D, Frick U. (1987) Interaction between man and shoe in running: considerations for a more comprehensive measurement approach. Int J Sports Med. 1987 Jun;8(3):196-202

Kroll W & Clarson PM (1978). Fractionated reflex time, resisted and unresisted fractionated reaction time under normal and fatigued conditions. In DM Landrers & RW. Christina (Eds), Psychology of Motor Behaviour and Sport 1977 (pp 106-129) Champaign ,IL: Human Kinetics.

Lieber RL (1992). Skeletal muscle response to injury. In: Skeletal muscle structure and function. John P Butler, Ed. Baltimore/Williams § Wilkins, 1992: 260-292

Luethi S, Stacoff A (1987).The influence of shoes on foot mechanics in running. Med. Sport Sci., 25:72-85.

Mann RA, Moran GT, Dogherty SE (1986). Comparative electromyography of the lower extremity in jogging, running and sprinting. The American Journal of sports Medicine 14 (6): 501-510.

Margaria R, Cavagna GA (1965). The mechanics of walking. J Physiol (Paris). Sep-Oct;57(5):655-6.

Martín PE, Morgan DW (1992). Biomechanical considerations for economical walking and running. Med. Sci. Sports Exerc. 24 (4):467-474.

Meinecke L., Disselhorst-Klug C., & Rau G. (2004): Crosstalk and Coactivation in Bipolar Surface EMG Data: A New Methodology for Detection, Discrimination and Quantification; in the 25th Congress of the International Society of Electrophysiological Kinesiology (ISEK), Boston, Massachusetts, June 2004, p. 87.

Milliron M, Cavanagh PR (1990). Sagittal plane kinematics of the lower extremity during distance running. In Biomechanics of distance running. Human Kinetics Books, Champaign Illinois.

Mundermann A, NiggBM, Humblew RN, Stefanyshyn DJ (2003). Foot orthotics affect lower extremity kinematics and kinetics during running. Cl Biom18: 254-262.

Nigg BM (1983). External force measurements with sport shoes and playing surfaces; in Nigg Kerr, Biomechanical aspects of sport shoes and playing surfaces 11-23 (University Printing, Calgary).

Nigg BM, Bahlsen HA, Denoth J, Luethi SM, Stacoff A (1986). Factors influencing kinetic and kinematic variables in tuning. In: Biomechanics of running shoes. BM Nigg (ed.). Pp 139-159. Champaign, IL: Human Kinetics Publishers.

Nigg BM, Wakeling JM (2001). Impact forces and muscle tuning: a new paradigm. Exerc Sport Sci Rev 29(1):37-41.

Nigg BM, Mundeermann A, Stefanyshyn DJ, Cole G, Stergiou P, Miller J (2003).The effect of material characteristics of shoe soles on muscle activation and energy aspects during running.J Biom 36: 569-575.

Novacheck TF (1998). The biomechanics of running. Gait & Posture 7: 77-95.

Perry J (1992). Gait analysis sistems in gait analysis: normal and pathological function. Thorofare, NJ: Slack 353-411.

Nordin M and Frankel VH (2004). Biomecanica de la rodilla. In: Biomecanica basica del sistema musculoesqueletico. McGraw Hill/Inteaméricana de Espana, S.A.U.

O'Connor KM, Hamill J (2005).The role of selected extrinsic foot muscles during running. Clin Biomech (2004) Jan;19(1):71-7.

Ramiro J, Ferranids R, Sánchez J, Alepuz R, Latorre P, Dejoz R, Candela F (1988). Evaluación de la técnica del calzado deportivo. Archivos Medicina del Deporte V (18): 161-168.

Reber L, Perry J, Pink M (1993). Muscular control of the ankle in running. Am J Sports Med 21 (6):805-810.

SENIAM (1999). European recommendations for surface electromyography.

Segesser B, Nigg BM (1993). Orthopedic and biomechanical concepts of sports shoe construction Sportverletz Sportschaden 7 (4) 150-162.

Shorteen MR (1993). The energetics of running and running shoes. J Biom 26 (1): 41-51.

Slocum DB, James SL (1968). Biomechanics of running. JAMA. 1968 Sep 9;205(11):721-8.

Staude G, Wolf W (1999). Objective motor response onset detection in surface myoelectric signals. Medical Engineering & Physics 21:449-467.

Testut L, Latarjet A (1971). Tratado de Anatomía Humana. Barcelona: Salvat editores.

Vaughan, CL (1984). Biomechanics of running. Crit Rev Biomed Eng 12:1-48

Wakeling JM, Von Tscharner V, Nigg BM, Stergiou P (2001). Muscle activity in the leg is tuned in response to ground reaction forces. J Appl Physiol Sep;91(3):1307-17.

Wakeling JM, Pascual S, Nigg B M (2002). Altering muscle activity in lower extremities by running with different shoes. Med. Sci. Sports Exerc. 34 (9): 1529-1532.

Winter DA (1979). Mechanical work, energy and power. In: Biomechanics of human movement. Pp 84-107. Toronto: John Wiley and Sons.

Winter DA (1990). Biomechanical and motor control of human movement, 2nd edn. New York:Wyley, 1990.

Winter DA, Fugelvand AJ, & Archer SE (1994). Crosstalk in surface electromyography: theoretical and practical estimates. Journal of Electromyography and Kynesiology 1994;4:15-26.

Wickiewiz TL, Roland R, Perry L, Powell BS, Edgerton R (1983). Muscle architecture of the human lower limb. Clinical Ortopaedics and Related Research 179: 275-283.

# Chapter 4

# Relationships Between Surface Electromyography and Strength During Isometric Ramp Contractions

Runer Augusto Marson

Additional information is available at the end of the chapter

## 1. Introduction

From the many joints exposed to muscle-skeletal injuries, the knee joint is the one that more suffers consuming in the daily life, for both athletes and non-athletes [1], once for the maintenance of the corporal stability, it is necessary for the muscles of this joint to be the strongest as possible [2]. Such strengthening may be obtained through an isometric force training [3], which range from numbers of repetitions up to weekly frequencies [4,5].

The hamstrings muscle group is objeto de estudo devido seu papel como músculo bi-articular, bem como a sua função na insuficiência mecânica [6]. This group is composed of the *semitendinosus* (ST), *semimembranosus* (SM) and *biceps femoris caput longum* (BFCL) all of which are active during knee flexion. The activity of these muscles is often examined using surface electromyography (sEMG) [7,8,9].

The efficiency of muscle contraction depends on factors such as the fiber cross-section, the number of muscle fibers, the degree of fiber stretching, the traction angle and the type of contraction required [5,10].

Isometric exercise is one of several forms of exercise used to develop muscle force in humans. Isometric contraction occurs without any appreciable change in muscle length, such that although there is tension in the muscle there is little muscle movement for most of the time, hence the term static contraction [6,11].

A important fact that be associated with a force output is the neuromuscular fatigue. This can under certain conditions be reflected in a decreased performance and/or the failure point at wich the muscle is no longer able to sustain the requeried force or work output level [12,13,14].

Research by [15] Dimitrova & Dimitrov (2002) related that Muscle fatigue is recognized as a decline in force, or failure to maintain the required or expected force. It may occur at any point from the nervous centers and conducting pathways to the contractile mechanism of muscle fibers.

Study by [16] Moritani & Yoshitake (1998)Such changes have been shown to be related to hydrogen ion and metabolite accumulation and to sodium and potassium ion concentration shifts. These changes would in turn affect the muscle excitation traction coupling including the muscle membrane properties and muscle action potential propagation, leading to sEMG manifestations of muscle fatigue distinct from mechanical manifestations.

The increase in amplitude of the sEMG signal as an empirical measure of localized muscle fatigue or as an indicator of muscle fatigue [9,17]. The RMS-sEMG values tended increase with decreasing force as a function of the number of repetitions [6] phenomenon that determines the neuromuscular fatigue process.

The active motor units also discharge with increasing speed to compensate for the fall in the force of contraction of the fatigued fibers [13,18].

The surface electromyography behavior at different force levels is of particular importance. This can be either achieved by performing multiple isometric contractions at various force levels or using ramp contractions.

A ramp contraction is defined as a progressive linear increase in force over time and relationships sEMG-force is linear or quadratic [19], and then, sEMG parameters and phsyiologicasl events used ramp contraction in investigation, as well, motor unit recruitments, force produce and gender influence [20].

Study by [19] Bilodeau et al (2003), [20] Pérot et al (1996) and [21] Stulen and DeLuca (1981) related the relationship of curve in ramp contraction were this behavior can be confirmed between of recruitment of large, type II muscles fibers, with a higher muscle action potential conduction velocity, is associated with an increase in the median frequency or mean power frequency values of the power spectrum of sEMG [22].

In the decade 80 researches showed that the ramp contraction procedure might be replaced by procedure comprising a number of distinct and constant force contraction. Ramp contractions involve the registration of sEMG while the strength performance gradually increases his or her level of effort up to maximal or submaximal levels. Although the latter procedure seems to be easier to use in some investigation, the ramp procedure has gained a wider acceptance since then. They have been extensively applied to examine muscle activation strategies as well as in new protocols of electromyography analysis. [19,23]

The purpose of the present study was to investigate the relationships of sEMG and time during isometric strength ramp contraction in the hamstrings muscle group. Hamstrings muscle group is composed of the *semitendinosus* (ST), *semimembranosus* (SM) and *biceps femoris caput longum* (BFCL) all of which are active during knee flexion.

## 2. Material and methods

### 2.1. Subject

Twenty female healthy adults (age 19.5 ± 0.8 yrs, body mass 63.4 ± 1.5 kg, height: 1.65 ± 0.05 m), without muscle skeletal disorders and similar anthropometric measurement, subject in this study. Subjects were all right leg dominant. All subjects signed a written informed consent. The study was approved by the AESA Ethics Committee protocol 344/10.

### 2.2. Equipment and electrode placement

Surface electromyography activity was collected by an eight-channel unit (EMG System do Brazil Ltda®) consisting of a band pass filter of 20–500Hz, an amplifier gain of 1000, and a common rejection mode ratio >100dB. All data were acquired and processed using a 16-bit analog to digital converter (EMG System do Brazil Ltda®), with a sampling frequency 1024 Hz. A channel of the acquisition system was enabled for the utilization of the load cell (SF01 - EMG System do Brazil Ltda®) having an output between 0 and 20mV and a range up to 5kN.

The biosignals from the *semitendinosus* (ST), *semimembranosus* (SM) and *biceps femoris caput longum* (BFCL) muscles were recorded with pairs of bipolar silver–silver chloride surface electrodes (10 mm electrode diameter, fixed inter-electrode distance of 20 mm). Following skin abrasion with an alcohol soaked cotton pad, electrodes were placed with the recommendation of Marson [6].

### 2.3. Ramp contractions

This protocol was had increase of maximal voluntary contraction (MVC) (10, 20 30 e 40%). The knee was flexion to 90º and isometric contractions were done by pulling on a cable fixed to the ankle which was kept at 90º relative to the longitudinal axis of the leg. The cable length was adjusted to the size of the subject's leg.

The load cell traction was performed initial with 10% MVC during 20s, immediately increased to 20% MVC during 20s. This characteristic was used until 40% of MVC.

Initially the participant with the knee flexed 90°, is a traction against the cell load corresponding to 10% maintaining that drift for 20 seconds. Immediately the participant was asked to traction 20% and so on for 30 and 40% MVC (Figure 1).

Continuous samples were collected these traction. These collections take place without the participants to rest between them. The RMS-sEMG values there is a change in load has been discarded (Figure 2).

### 2.4. Signal processing

The sEMG signals were amplified with gain 1000. The analog channel band pass was set to 20-500 Hz and the sampling rate for analog-to-digital conversion was 1024 Hz.

For analyses time-domain the ramp contractions, sEMG-RMS value, were calculated from a 200 millisecond (ms) window at each the following force levels: 10%, 20%, 30% e 40% of MVC.

For signal processing of each isometric ramp contractions was used routine development by Matlab® and OriginLab©.

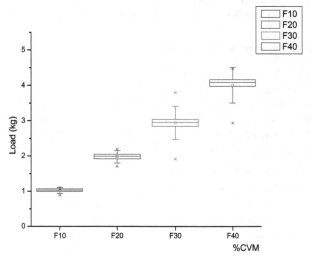

**Figure 1.** Box chart of mean,standard deviation and percentile (25,75) in 10% (F10), 20% (F20), 30%, (F30) and 40% (F40) of CVM

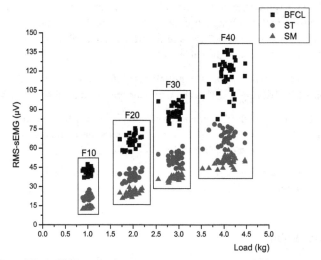

**Figure 2.** Relation of RMS-sEMG (µV) value versus CVM (kg). The rectangular box is the 10% (F10), 20% (F20), 30%, (F30) and 40% (F40) of CVM.

## 3. Results and discussion

Isometric exercises have shown a diversity of results regarding the strength gain and with it major changes have occurred regarding its inclusion within methods of strength training. This type of training is applied, mostly in clinics specializing in rehabilitation, physiotherapy and sports training centers aimed at improving muscle and joint injuries [8].

One of the most difficult physical qualities to be worked on is the strength, because a mistake in any application can lead to unpleasant consequences, such as stretching and muscle contractures. So the force is a physical quality that shows a vector quantity, it has magnitude and direction. The vectors are displayed graphically by a line of action, showing the direction and an attachment point of great importance for daily tasks as well as sports performance.

In the isometric there is a consensus response to an increase in sEMG as to alter some characteristic muscle joint as the increase in signal amplitude [13,24,25,26] changes the length and range of motion [27] and temperature [28,29,30].

Classic research shown that there is not always a tendency for this linearity. Research by [31] DeLuca & Lawrence (1983) studied the electromyographic behavior of the biceps brachii, deltoid and 1st dorsal interosseous fadigantes isometric contractions. They concluded that for the interosseous muscle was an almost linear relationship, but further analysis showed a characteristic polynomial 2nd order, the same is true for the biceps and deltoid muscles that showed a remarkable non-linearity of your data.

Studies [32] Clamann & Broecker (1979) who analyzed the triceps brachii, biceps, adductor pollicis and 1st interosseous, and [33] Woods & Bigland-Ritchie (1983) who analyzed the triceps brachii, biceps, adductor pollicis and soleus, showed that the electromyographic signal amplitude as a function of force applied to the interosseous muscle and adductor pollicis was always an almost linear relationship to the muscles and biceps, triceps and soleus this relationship was not linear, unless an exception of biceps brachii this relationship was almost linear [32].

Recent research report the nonlinear characteristic between amplitude of depolarization of motor units related to time and muscle strength [11,34]. This non-linear increase was also observed in this present study (Figure 3) in isometric ramp contraction test during time performance. The data presented in a slow onset, over time it has a rapid and finally back to grow slowly of sEMG amplitude.

According [35] Miyashita et al. (1981) and [11] Marson (2010) acting with incremental the amplitude of the electromyographic signal has an almost linear function of time to begin the individual fatigued. After the onset of muscular fatigue process the signal begins to have an increase predominantly curvilinear.

The electromyographic signal has quite often been used as a mean of assessment of muscle fatigue [17]. The increase in amplitude (Figure 3) of the EMG signal as an empirical measure of localized muscle fatigue or as an indicator of muscle fatigue [15].

Research by [15] Dimitrova & Dimitrov (2002) related that muscle fatigue is recognized as a decline in force, or failure to maintain the required or expected force. It may occur at any

point from the nervous centers and conducting pathways to the contractile mechanism of muscle fibers.

Study by [16] Moritani & Yoshitake (1998) such changes have been shown to be related to hydrogen ion and metabolite accumulation and to sodium and potassium ion concentration shifts. These changes would in turn affect the muscle excitation traction coupling including the muscle membrane properties and muscle action potential propagation, leading to sEMG manifestations of muscle fatigue distinct from mechanical manifestations.

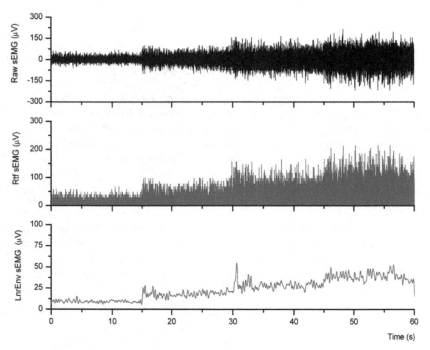

**Figure 3.** The raw sEMG (Raw sEMG), retificated (Rtf sEMG) and Linear envelope (LnrEnv sEMG) during ramp isometric contraction. Example figure.

The EMG amplitude increased progressively with increasing force in all muscles. The similar behavior was expressed as a percent of the RMS-sEMG value obtained during the brief pre-fatigue MVCs.

The data was fitting non linear by equation (1)

$$f(x) = \frac{A_1 - A_2}{1 + e^{(x_n - x_0)/d_x}} + A_2 \tag{1}$$

The $f(x)$ represents the data set in the RMS $x$-axis (time), A1 is the initial value of the RMS collected, the final value of $A2$ RMS, $x0$ is the point of inflection of the sigmoidal fit curve, i.e., the instant that there is a change from convex to concave curve which is found by the coordinate $(x0,y0)$, where $y0$ and found by equation (2). Since the coordinate $y0$ is found the value of $x0$ on the time axis.

$$y_0 = \frac{A1 + A2}{2} \qquad (2)$$

The $dn$ parameter is found using equation (3)

$$d_n = \frac{x_n - x_0}{\log(A_1 - A_2) - 1/y_n - A_2} \qquad (3)$$

The $dn$ parameter is the value obtained for each of the coordinate values $x$ and $y$. After obtaining all the values of $dn$ is done an average, and this is adopted with the value of the constant parameter $dx$.

Several studies report that the increase in the electrical function of time, fatiguing contractions, is characterized by the linearity between these data. Methods to assess muscle fatigue by surface electromyography are elaborated upon this predominance [11,34,36].

This nonlinear increase was also observed in this present study in ramp isometric contractions test. The data presented in the early slow growth over the same time is a rapid increase and eventually grow back slowly. With these data in hand a mathematical model was developed, based on the characteristic sigmoidal or logistic curve (Figure 4-6).

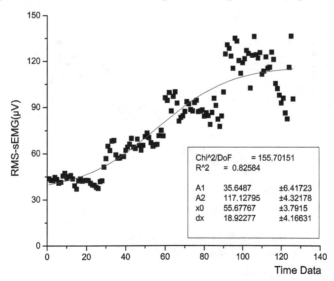

**Figure 4.** Relationship, adjust and parameter nonlinear of RMS-sEMG value. BFCL example.

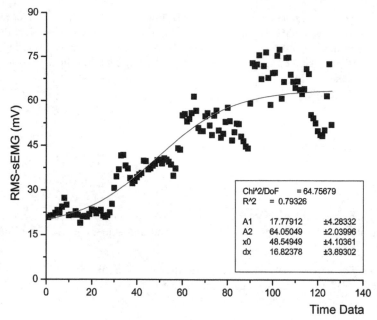

**Figure 5.** Relationship, adjust and parameter nonlinear of RMS-sEMG value. ST example.

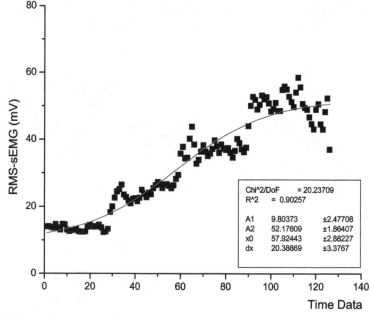

**Figure 6.** Relationship, adjust and parameter nonlinear of RMS-sEMG value. SM example.

The adjustment was made by equation 1. To verify that this setting was close to actual data (data collected) was analyzed the coefficient of determination ($r^2$) between the actual data and the adjusted data, where the $r^2$ values greater than 0.80.

According to [37] Enoka and Stuart (1992), [35] Miyashita et al. (1981) in incremental overhead fatiguing exercise with the amplitude of the electromyographic signal has an almost linear function of time until the individual begins to fatigue. After the onset of muscle fatigue process the signal begins to increase a predominantly curvilinear [38].

This characteristic presented in this mathematical adjustment points that are side left of the parameter $x0$ which is the turning point of the concavity of the sigmoidal curve. This behavior provides a characterization of possible fatigue neuromuscular isometric ramp contractions.

## 4. Conclusion

Investigations have been concerned in the restricted use of the isometric contraction ramp during a single, non-fatiguing, and linearly increasing contraction force variation at short intervals, it is suggested that where the isometric ramp contractions can provide higher resolution in the entire spectrum force, less time required for data acquisition electromyography, and less susceptible to fatigue than contractions step. It is possible, however, that whereas the ramp and contraction power spectrum characteristic of the control strategies can incorporate various engine and comparing the dynamic and isometric contractions isokinetic step.

This present study revealed that the relationship between electromyography, force and time has characteristic sigmoidal. This demonstrates that the initial charges in a relationship are slowly increasing, but at intermediate loads this increase is more rapid and exponential. However, this behavior the load end presents a decrease in the rate of increase and maintenance of a depolarization of motor units at the end of execution of the isometric ramp contraction.

This sigmoidal relationship data is well described in the equation proposed for modeling (curve fitting) of hamstring muscle electromyographic signal analyzed, which is presented the start point ($A1$), the constant in equation ($dx$), the turning point the concavity of the curve ($x0$) and peak ($A2$) to be kept in mathematical adjustment of the curve in relation to actual curve acquired.

In summary, the results of this study indicate that RMS values of the hamstrings muscles tend to increase nonlinear whereas force with the number of isometric ramp contractions performed.

## 5. Future directions

Since these responses are characteristic of neuromuscular fatigue, the test described here may be useful for identifying muscle fatigue in ramp isometric contraction test. With this feature researches, in future studies, propose mathematical models to identify the turning point of the concavity of the sigmoid adjustment for the analysis and identification of the electromyographic fatigue. Therefore, in order to develop a new protocol for the identification of fatigue could be observed electromyographic initial characteristics of the sigmoid curve which is a slow increase over time data, which has an exponential characteristic. With these parameters can ascertain exponential models as the inflection point of the curve for possible identification of neuromuscular fatigue.

Understanding the importance of digital signal processing, in this case the surface electromyographic signal, the mathematical adjustment (mathematical modeling), presents itself as a tool to direct future research related to bioengineering, which may direct future investigations from the area of instrumentation to the development of new systems of man-machine synchronization.

## Author details

Runer Augusto Marson

*Laboratory of Biomechanics and Kinesiology, Sport Center, Federal University of Ouro Preto, Minas Gerais, Brazil*

*Laboratory of Biomechanics, Research Institute of Physic Capacity of the Army, Rio de Janeiro, Brazil*

## 6. References

[1] Zatsiorsky, V.M. 2000. *Biomechanics in Sport Performance: improvement and injury prevention.* 2000. Oxford: Blackwell Science LTD.

[2] Lippert, L. 2011. *Clinical kinesiology and anatomy,* 5th ed. Philadelphia: F. A. Davis Company.

[3] Kumar, S. 2004. *Muscle Strength.* Danver: CRC Press LLC.

[4] Verkhoshansky, Y. V. 2004. *Special Strength Training: a pratical manual for coaches.* Moscow: MOCKBA.

[5] Garfinkel S; Cafarelli E.1992. Relative changes in maximal force, EMG, and muscle cross-sectional area after isometric training. *Medice and Science in Sports and Exercise.* 24: 1220-27.

[6] Marson, R.A.; Gonçalves, M., 2003. Electromyographic behavior of the biceps femoris (caput longum) and semitendinosus muscles in the isometric contraction test. Brazilian *J. Morphol. Sci..* 20:55-7.

[7] Solomonow M, Krogsgaard M. Sensorimotor control of knee stability: a review. *Scan J Med Sci Sports* 2001;11:64–80.

[8] Kellis,E; Katis, A. Reliability of EMG power-spectrum and amplitude of the semitendinosus and biceps femoris muscles during ramp isometric contractions. *J. Electromyograph Kinesiol* 18 (2008) 351–358.

[9] Marson Ra, Gonçalves M (2001) Comportamento eletromiográfico do músculo biceps femoris (caput longum) submetido a exercício isométrico. In: *Anais do IX Congresso Brasileiro de Biomecânica.* Gramado (RS), Brazil, 29 May-1 June. pp. 289-293.

[10] Garfinkel S; Cafarelli E.1992. Relative changes in maximal force, EMG, and muscle cross-sectional area after isometric training. *Med. Sci. Sports Exerc.* 24: 1220-27.

[11] Marson, R.A. Identificación de la fatiga electromiográfica en contracciones isométricas crecientes. *Lecturas Educación Física y Deportes*, 15:146 - Julio de 2010.

[12] Moritani T.; Nagata, A.; Devries, H.A.; Muro, M., 1981. Critical power as a measure of physical work capacity and anaerobic threshold. *Ergonomics*.24:339-50.

[13] BASMAJIAN JV; Deluca CJ. 1985. *Muscle Alive:* Their Function Revealed by Electromyography. Baltimore:Willians & Wilkins. p.201-222.

[14] Dimitrova Na; Dimitrov, GV. 2003. Interpretation of EMG changes with fatigue: facts, pitfalls, and fallacies. *J. Electromyograph Kinesiol*, 13:13-36.

[15] Dimitrova, Na; Dimitrov, GV. 2002. Amplitude-related characteristics of motor unit and M-wave potentials during fatigue. A simulation study using literature data on intracellular potential changes found in vitro. *J. Electromyograph Kinesiol*, 12:339-349.

[16] Moritani, T; Yoshitake, Y. 1998 ISEK Congress Keynote Lecture:The use of electromyography in applied physiology. *J Electromyograph Kinesiol*, 8:363-81.1998.

[17] Moritani, T.; Muro, M.; Nagata, A., 1986. Intramuscular and surface electromyogram changes during muscle fatigue. *J. Applied Physiol.* 60:1179-85.

[18] Petrofsky Js, Lind AR (1980) The influence of temperature on the amplitude and frequency components of the EMG during brief and sustained isometric contractions. Eur. *J. Appl. Physiol.* 44, 189-200.

[19] Bilodeau M, Schindler-Ivens S, Williams DM, Chandran R, Sharma SS. EMG frequency changes with increasing force and during fatigue in the quadriceps femoris muscle of men and women. *J Electromyogr Kinesiol* 2003;13:83–92.

[20] Pérot, C.; André, L.; Dupont, L.; Vanhouttle, C. Relative contributions of the long and shorts head of the biceps brachii during simple or dual isometrics tasks. *J. Electromyograph. Kinesiol.*, 6:3-11, 1996.

[21] Stulen, F.; Deluca, C.J. Frequency parameters of the myoeletric signal as a measure of muscle conduction value. IEEE Trans. *Biomed. Eng.* BME, 28:515-23, 1981.

[22] Dupont, L.; Gamet, D.; Pérot, C. Motor unit recruitment and EMG power spectra during ramp contraction of a bifunctional muscle. *J. Electromyograph. Kinesiol*, 10:217-24, 2000.

[23] Sanchez Jh, Solomonow M, Baratta Rv, D'ambrosia R. Control strategies of the elbow antagonist muscle pair during two types of increasing isometric contractions. *J Electromyograph Kinesiol* 1993;3:33–40.

[24] FarinA, D.; Holobar, A. Gazzoni, M.; Zazula, D.; Merletti, R.; Enoka, R.M. Adjustments differ among low-threshold motor units during intermittent isometric contraction. *J. Neurophysiol*, 101:350-359, 2009.

[25] Hug, F.; Nordez, A.; Guèvel, A. Can the electromyographic fatigue threshold be determined from superficial elbow flexors musclesduring an isometric sigle-joint task? Eur. *J. Appl. Physiol*, 101:193-201, 2009.

[26] James, C.R.; Scheuermann, B.W.; Smith, M.P. Effect of two neuromuscular fatigue protocols on landing performance. *J. Electromyograph Kinesiol.*, 20:667-675, 2010.

[27] Bandy, W.; Hanten, W.P. Changes in torque and electromyography activity of the quadriceps femoris muscles following isometric training. *Physical Therapic*, Danver, n.73, p.455-65, 1993

[28] Petrofsky, J.S.; Lind, A. R. The influece of temperature on the amplitude and frequecy components of the EMG during brief and sustained isometric contractions. *Eur J Applied Physiol*, Berlin, n. 44, p. 189-200, 1980.

[29] Kimura, T.; Hamada, T.; Ueno, L.M.; Moritani, T. Changes on contractile properties and neuromuscular propagation evaluated by simultaneous mechanomyogram and electromyogram during experimentally induce hypothermia. *J. Electromyograph Kinesiology*, 13: 433-440, 2003

[30] Farina, D.; Arendt-Nielsen, L.; Graven-Nielsen, T. Effect of temperature on spike-triggedere average torque and electrophysiological properties of low-threshold motor units. *J. Appl. Physiol.* 99:197-203, 2005.

[31] Deluca, C.J,; LAWRENCE, J.H. Effect of muscle on the EMG signal-force relationship. *J Applied Physiol*, Bethesda, v.13, p.77, 1983.

[32] Clamann, H.P.; Broecker, K.T. Relation beteween force and fatigability pad and pate skeletal muscles in man. *Am J Phys Medicine*, Baltimore, v.58, p.70-85, 1979.

[33] Woods J.J; Bigland-RitchiE, B. Linear and non-linear surface EMG/force relationships in human muscles. *Am. J Phys Medicine*, Baltimore, v.62, p.287, 1983.

[34] Marson, R.A. Study of muscular fatigue by EMG analysis during isometric exercise. In: ISSNIP *Biosignal and Biorobotics*,Conference, 2011.

[35] Miyashita, M.; Kanehisa, H.; Nemoto, I. EMG related to anaerobic threshold. *J Sports Med Physical Fitness*, London, v.21, p.209-17, 1981.

[36] DeVries HA (1968) Method for evaluation of muscle fatigue and endurance from electromyography fatigue curves. *Am. J. Physiol. Med.* 47, 125-135.

[37] Enoka, R.M.; Stuart, D.G. Neurobiology of muscle fatigue. *J. Applied Physiol.* 72:1631-48, 1992.

[38] Yao, W.; Figlevand, A.J.; Enoka, R.M. Motor-units synchronization increases EMG amplitude and decreases force steadiness of simulated contractions. *J. Neurophysiol.* 83:441-52, 2000.

# Chapter 5

# Influence of Different Strategies of Treatment Muscle Contraction and Relaxation Phases on EMG Signal Processing and Analysis During Cyclic Exercise

Leandro Ricardo Altimari, José Luiz Dantas, Marcelo Bigliassi,
Thiago Ferreira Dias Kanthack, Antonio Carlos de Moraes and Taufik Abrão

Additional information is available at the end of the chapter

## 1. Introduction

For a long time we work with muscular activity, trying to answer questions related to fatigue, muscle activity and other issues related to neuromuscular system. In this way we started to use the electromyography (EMG) as a tool to achieve better results in our studies, since it appeared to us as a truthful method to access the muscle activity inside a lot of perspectives we had been working with.

In this chapter we will try to bring some research results that we found on the GEPESINE laboratory in the last couple of years about regarding the EMG analysis. Firstly there are relevant issues that arise during the use of EMG as a tool in others works. It is not hard to find studies that use EMG signal as a way to measure the muscle activity [1-3], muscle fatigue [4] and also in studies involving healthy issues [5]. Most of those studies try to access the activity or fatigue slope of the muscle during some motor task, mostly trying to access performance or just to categorize an activity according to the muscle(s) accessed. The real problem is that most of those studies use isometric movements or even isokinetic, leaving a remarkable problem for the researchers who decide to work with dynamic contractions, once the available protocols are most based on and suitable isometric studies.

We have decided to take a different look to the process on how to treat the EMG signal and how to analyze it. For instance, in order to have a more trustful signal, founds in literature recommend filtering, smoothing the raw and also rectifying the signal, which the last step does not affect the signal power. However, the filtered root mean square (RMS) signal could not be the best way to pre-process the EMG signal. Other current concern, in EMG signal pre-processing, is about the use of the total signal against evaluation only the burst-time segments of the signal. Those concerns are explained and analyzed along this chapter. In an epistemological language, we take a more critic look into the EMG signal processing. We hope the reader also to have the same look, not only into the results and conclusions, but also, into methods and thoughts, since the intention herein is not to bring an irrefutable true, but the real intention is to discuss and point out valuable arguments for the reader in order to he/she thinks about it by himself or herself, and apply it properly.

## 2. Theory

### 2.1. The importance of electromyography in cyclic exercises

Cyclic exercises correspond to modalities such as bicycle, running, walking and swimming. Inside those we can already imagine a lot of different sports with a great repercussion over the media, a few examples include: street bike, mountain bike and tour, like the famous Tour of France; marathon, 400 meters, race walking and putting in just one thing, the triathlon. You may notice that the swimming sports are not exemplified above, it's because it is still hard to access the muscle activity through electromyography in those sports due to the environment where they happens. This discussion was set aside for our future work

So, keeping in mind that some of the most important sports have a cyclic dynamic as characterization, for the evolution of them, new technologies need to be able to help the coaches and physical trainers. Nowadays individual time-trial sports are reaching world records that we would never imagine, and every new record is followed by a technology behind it helping in training or even during the task if is not prohibited. To be able to access the muscle activity with a good reliability in different moments of the exercise could give us the weak and the strong moments of one athlete during the task, and allow us to create the better strategy and also create new training cycles that can improve the weakness. It is worth noting the electromyography is useful to access not only muscle activity -- in order to enhance the performance in sports --, but also be deployed in exercises evaluation aiming healthy improvement.

### 2.2. Time and frequency domain

Talk about frequency domain is talk about: how many times a event occurs in a time space, in this way, to use this component we need transform the signal in different points presented in a frequency spectrum capable to show us the energy of cue obtained in the determined muscle. This energy in the most part of the time appears represented in some bands, where your intensity and duration has more amplitude. To find and use the spectrum, we must find a source that gives us the possibility to produce this figure, when sometimes the Fast Fourier Transform proves as algorithm in a simple calculus to find discrete signals. A series of recommendations are proposed to this technique, since the establishment of sample number,  duration intervals, window apply and many aspects as signal stationary  is a complicated thing to deal with, which leads us to use a wavelet transform, more appropriate to cyclic activities as cycling and running for example [6-9].

Independently of technique used we should get some variable from this analyses to compare, relate or make our considerations, in this case, the most common variable toke from frequency domain is the median frequency, representative of fatigue aspect in the muscular activity from decrease of conduct fibers velocity, is exactly the point that divided the spectrum in two equal parts and gives us a good representation of reduction in the force produced.

Time domain is used when the intention is to achieve the contractibility of the muscle, meaning that as stronger the signal the most number of motor units are been activated. The most common variable used inside this domain is the Root Mean Square (RMS) [9]. To get this variable some procedures are required, like the filtration, rectification and smoothing, those will be better explained later. Just like the frequency domain, a correct time window is necessary and follows the frequency domain also when talking about the use of wavelet transform.

## 2.3. Treating the EMG signal

Now you already know about how the domains work and how to use them for different analysis depending on the applications necessity. During the subchapter "Analysis of the EMG signal" we hope it became clear that we have some procedures until the real signal is accessed, especially without noises. The raw signal can already give us some information, like the muscle innervations or even the change in the signal size. Depending of the intention, these qualitative variables can be very useful. An easy and good way to simple control some noises when there is no intention of further computer treatment to remove it, is to be sure to have a good baseline, meaning that the line that should appear at the EMG signal must be as close as it can to zero when the muscle with the electrode connected is not in contraction. That doesn't mean that when the muscle starts to contract the signal that will appear will only be from the muscle activity, especially in dynamic contractions. There are three main differences in noises on static contractions and dynamic ones, they are: the non-stationarity of the signal for the constant contraction and relaxing of the muscle, the change of the electrode distance relative to the origin of the action potential and the changes in the conductivity of the tissues properties [10].

A better way to understand what a noise is, is looking at it, the figure 1 under is an EMG signal with a closer look in the burst moment. Notice that the areas surrounded with black circles have a peculiar difference, it has a horizontal straight shaped line, which means that those parts don't have a corresponding negative part, and so, it is considered a noise. Of course in this same image you can find some more of those, not only the surrounded ones, but the intention here is only to show how a noise appears inside an EMG signal.

When the signal appears to us in the computer screen those details are impossible to see without a zoom look. So, lets talk now about how the treatments can influence in the signal value.

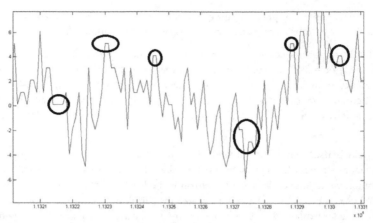

**Figure 1.** Noises in the EMG signal

Note the figure 2 under, pay even more attention to the baseline in the raw signal, it is close to zero because it almost creates a straight line, considering that the muscle in this case is the vastus lateralis in a bike-like exercise, we can imagine that in the beginning of the exercise he is not much triggered, probably because the recto femuralis is doing almost all the job, but as time goes and also the exercise, its starts to have stronger signal, so we can imagine that the other muscles, like the recto femuralis is entering in fatigue process, so the vasto lateralis as a co-worker has to get part of this charge in order to maintain the exercise, that is the kind of qualitative analyze that was told before, without even knowing the values numbers, we can visually access an ideia about the use of vasto lateralis in a cicliergometer exercise.

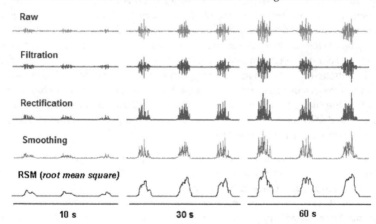

**Figure 2.** EMG signal process recommended. Green: The raw signal, no treatment was applied until this moment; Red: Filtrated signal, a limit was created for the signal, excluding everything out of it; Blue: Rectified signal, all negative values were transformed in positive ones and added; Purple: the smoothed signal, a linear enveloped was created and the extreme parts of the signal was excluded; Black: The RMS values after all the treatments.

With the intention of clearing the EMG signal, and make it more reliable and truthful, some computer processes are used before analyzes, they are: Filtration, Rectification and Smoothing. The image below shows the same signal from raw until the smoothed in order to obtain the RMS values for the vastus lateralis muscle in an exercise in 100% of the maximal watts in a cicloergometer during 60 seconds. Those process, expecially the Filtration and the Smoothing has the purpose of giving us the possibility to evaluate only the signal coming from the muscular contraction, without mechanical or electromagnetic interferences [2,11].

## 2.3.1. Signal filtering

In a first moment the filtration occurs when the signal is been collected. With the objective to avoid interferences the EMG signal passes through a 50 to 60 Hz filter (notch filter), if it's necessary. This filter already starts rejecting the frequency band of 60 Hz once that in this band is where the ambient interferences like pressure appear, arrangement or closer apparatus. In a second moment, the EMG signal must pass through a pass-band; this pass-band frequency must be decided by the analyzer, once it can depend on the intentions of the study. Normally, this frequency is fixed between 20 and 450 Hz, because normally 80% of the muscular energy is concentrated [12-13]. But, as said before, it is a free choice for the user, once that this frequency can differ from muscle to muscle, so, it's important for the user to know exactly the band of the muscle that is been assessed to make sure that the pass-band will cut off only the signal that doesn't belong to that muscle, and at the same time guarantee as precisely as it can that it won't let noises get inside the signal. Basically, it limits the signal inside a previous decided range to maintain it inside the muscle activation site.

The visual difference between the raw and the filtrated signal can be really hard to notice especially when the collected process is well cared, however, if we take a rigorous look to both of them, the difference will appear to our eyes, but remembering that the main reason of using those treatments is to obtain the quantitative values of the signal.

## 2.3.2. Signal rectification

This procedure has the purpose to turn all the signal values integrative, submitting them to the cut of all negative values, that means, to delete the values that are under the baseline, or to turn all this negative values to positive adding the values, making them integrative. The second option is more recommended if the intention is to achieve the total muscle signal, if you cut off the negative part, half of the signal will be lost, so turning all of them positive is a more used and more interesting when it comes to final results. This procedure doesn't affect the signal noises like the filtration and the smoothing, which will be explained in sequence. However it is still recommended and made part of the studies involving this chapter, so it's important for the reader to know how we used and what it means.

This procedure is simple, and it can be easily understood by the figure above. Note that until the filtration moment the signal had both positive and negative side in the burst moments, taking the baseline as a zero mark, and once that the signal was rectified it became not only positive, but also increased the positive side size, that mean that we didn't exclude the negative part, we added it to the positive side. If the reader wants to know how the same signal without the adding of the negative values would be, you just have to take the filtrated signal and cut the down part, always considering the baseline as a zero mark. Look at the figure 3 under and try to make a qualitative analyze of the two methods.

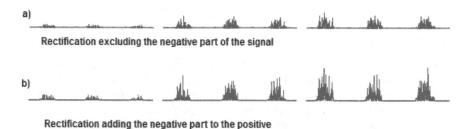

Figure 3. a) Half-wave rectification: rectification excluding the negative part of signal amplitude; b) Full-wave rectification: aggregating the negative part (reducing the ripple) of EMG signal.

Notice that for a visual analysis excluding the negative parte can bring an error, it's hard to say that the three last bursts of the red signal are different from the three before it, but in the blue signal is much easier to assume that. Thus in the first one I could say that the muscle had reached his maximal power, while in the second I could not make the same affirmation.

### 2.3.3. Signal smoothing

The Smoothing and the filtration have some similar parameters, mostly because both have the intention of taking out the extremes, the parts that are considering noises. Smoothing creates a linear envelope in the signal, leaving only a center part of the signal. The mainly difference between the smoothing and the filtration, is that filtration take in account the muscle activation range, and the smoothing the signal obtained itself. If the filter is strong enough or considered really good, it can even make the smoothing unnecessary. However, it's recommended to use both, especially in cyclic dynamic contractions, that as we already saw, have a bigger chance to have noises interferences. Looking at the Figure again, the smoothed signal is also really easy to realize, it creates visually a much cleaner signal, creating almost a line, which means, it excludes the extremes, leaving only the signal that is considered the muscle activation signal.

### 2.4. Burst and silence

During the obtainment of the EMG signal we can separate two parts of it, the Silence and the Burst, as showed in the figure 4.

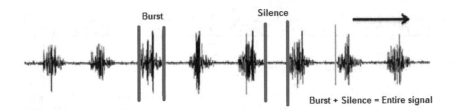

**Figure 4.** Burst and silence moments in an electromyography signal during a Wingate test in a cicloergometer. The break between the blue lines show a burst moment and the break between the red lines is the silence moment. Unification of Burst and Silence generates the full signal.

The Burst moment is the muscle contraction moment, easily noticed by the sudden break in the baseline, and so, the Silence moment is when no contraction is occurring, so the signal stays at zero, or at least should stay, as said before in the treatment discussions. That's another important reason to maintain a baseline close to zero; it is easier to separate the onset and the end of the Burst from the Silence moment. When a signal is collected it's normal to treat it as an Entire signal, which means that it takes to account both Burst and Silence moments of the signal. The figure showed above is from the recto femoral muscle in a cyclic exercise in a cicloergometer during a Wingate test. As expected in this kind of exercise, it is found a lot of Burst and Silence moments, differing from isometric exercises for example, that would appear only a Burst moment, which would lose strength as time goes by for the fatigue process.

The problem is the use of the entire signal, or only the Burst moments, taking into account that if the intention is to read only the muscle activity it can be assumed that should be used only the Burst moment once that a cyclic exercise will have a lot of Silence moments, and this could make the final results to become smaller, to decrease the meaning. Thus, to know if the Silence moment affects the final results in time and frequency domains variables is of great importance for the researchers that works especially with cyclic exercises. That is one of the problems that will be further discussed on this chapter.

## 2.5. Time windows

The term "time windows" is used to determine the size of the cuts that will be made in the EMG signal for further analyzes. The most normal is to use the 1 second window, and in case of short tasks it can easily be done once that the signal is short and it is easy to separate the total task time in 1 second parts. However, for longer tasks it can be really difficult for the researcher to separate a signal of 10 minutes in 600 windows of 1 second each for example. Thus, a study from [14] brought that to use a 5 second window and a 1 second in a cyclic exercise can provide the same result of muscle activity for further analyzes, providing for the EMG researchers an excitement about using the method in long tasks. To bring a better example, the figure 5 under shows us a signal and how it would be analyzed if it was cut in one second windows.

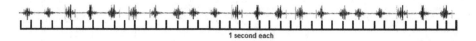

1 second each

**Figure 5.** An EMG signal divided in 1 second time windows.

In the same signal, the next image has the cuts made in five seconds windows (Figure 6). The biggest importance about using a bigger window is not just because it would be hard for the researcher to divide the signal, but also because some routines that treat the signal don`t accept too much windows to process.

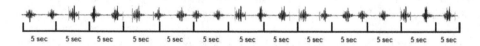

5 sec    5 sec    5 sec    5 sec    5 sec    5 sec    5 sec    5 sec    5 sec    5 sec    5 sec    5 sec    5 sec

**Figure 6.** The same EMG signal of Figure 5, now divided in 5 seconds windows.

## 3. Methodology

### 3.1. Influence of the treatments (First study)

The Signal processing in EMG is a complex matter to adopt in determined studies, in several times the signal process used is based on the mainly recommendations and the needs of researcher, but sometimes the instructions are not so clear and are not based in studies that contemplate the new tendencies in contemporary researches. However, the main objective of this chapter is to show the great possibility of using the different treatments to find the same outcome of an EMG signal, using many combinations of process (filtration, rectification and smoothing) in a variable of time domain (RMS) and discover if bursts are capable to interfere in the final result of a dynamic exercise in high intensity that is more capable to induce great noises. In that way, we keep our efforts in test these intriguing questions about the signal processing in EMG with a considerable method to involve the main exercise capable of producing the high amount of noises in the signal and test in this sequence the differences in use several proceedings in dynamic exercise (cycling). To introduce this perspective we assessed in a first period 20 men (27,5 ± 4,1 years old; 83,1 ± 8,2 kg; 184,5 ± 4,5 cm), healthy and active physically.

Briefly the subjects passed for a session of familiarization in the protocols and the instruments of the test, basically to know the cycle simulator and find/keep adjusts in bench and foot pedals. In the next step the men did a maximal incremental test (MIT) until exhaustion to determine the maximal work load (MWL). The information obtained in MIT was used to find the intensity of effort in constant load tests (CLT) in three different intensities in severe domain: 80% MWL, 100% MWL and 110% MWL, see figure 7 for better understanding. The different intensities in severe domain were chosen with the intention to allow us to make affirmations including all domains. Each subject was tested in the same hour of day to minimize the effects of the circadian variations.

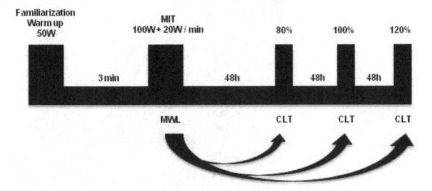

**Figure 7.** Illustrative representation of the first study, involving signal treatments for RMS obtainment.

Initially it was realized the MWL with initial load in 100W and 20W of increments each minute until voluntary exhaustion, remain a cadence of 70 revolutions per minute (rpm). The MWL was preceded of a warm-up with a load of 50W, with a period of three minutes, follow by three minutes in rest. The MWL was defined as a higher work load maintained for 30 seconds at least, this was assumed so we could make sure to achieve the MWL and not the peak load.

From the information obtained in the MWL, the subjects were oriented to realize three constant load tests (CLT) in different intensities, these being: submaximal (80%MWL), maximal (100%) and supramaximal (110%). Every test was realized in a cyclesimulator (Computrainer™, Racer Mate®, USA). The tests occur with at least 48 hours between then. The CLT was preceded of three minutes of warm-up with 50W, followed by three minutes of rest. After that the tests occur until exhaustion. The subjects were instructed to keep their cadence in 90 rpm, could not pedal less than that, and the test was interrupted when the subjects reported voluntary exhaustion or showed inability to keep the cadence stipulated on the test. The verbal encouragement was used.

The EMG signal was obtained during all period of realization in CLT using an electromyography with 16 channels, model MP150™ (Biopac System®, USA) with a sampling rate of 2000 samples/second, in agreement with ISEK [15]. Before the beginning of each CLT, the subjects were submitted to asepsis and curettage. The electrodes used were active and bipolar, model TSD 150™ (BIOPAC Systems®, USA), with distance among electrodes fixed in two centimeters, putted above superficial muscles of quadriceps femoral of right leg: vastus lateralis (VL), vastus medialis (VM) and rectus femoris (RF), following the standard of SENIAM [12], as showed by the white circles on the figure 8.

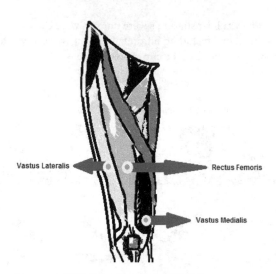

**Figure 8.** Electrode position used; SENIAM recommendations [12].

The relation of rejection common mode was >95dB and the limits of entrance of established signal in ± 5 mV. The reference electrode was positioned in the right elbow (lateral epicondyle). To capture and process the signal was used the software AcqKnowledge 3.8.1™ (BIOPAC Systems®, USA) and the software MatLab 7.0 (Mathworks®, South Natick, MA, USA).

The EMG signal was treated to obtain the RMS (root mean square) values in time windows with five seconds in the first minute of the test in different intensities. The first twenty seconds of each signal were discarded with the intention to avoid possible inertial influences. After that, it was used proceedings recommended to exclude artifacts and noises from EMG signal, divided in conditions: raw (R), Filtration (F), Filtration + smoothing (FS), filtration + smoothing + rectification (FSR). The filtration was done using a pass-band digital filter Butterworth with frequencies of 20 and 500 Hz. The smoothing process was done through a mobile mean with three points. The process of rectification was done considering all signals, without discards of negative part. The table 1 present the mean values of the load used in the constant load test in 80, 100 and 110% of MWL and the respective times to exhaustion.

| Condition | Load (W) | Time (s) |
|:---------:|:--------:|:--------:|
| CLT 80%  | $212.6 \pm 23.5^a$ | $1070.0 \pm 250.5^a$ |
| CLT 100% | $268.5 \pm 33.6^b$ | $282.3 \pm 75.5^b$ |
| CLT 110% | $301.5 \pm 31.7^c$ | $110.3 \pm 22.3^c$ |

Note: different letters show significant differences between loads and times to exhaustion, ($P<0.05$).

**Table 1.** Loads and times to exhaustion (mean and standard deviation) on constant load tests in 80, 100 and 110% of MWL.

## 3.2. Influence of the burst and silence in treatment of EMG signal (Second Study)

To test the possibility of bursts get in the way of an EMG signal and change the final outcome, we used a similar method, assessing 27 healthy students (14 men, age = 28,2 ± 2,7 years and 13 women, age = 23,2 ± 2,7 years). The test proposed was the Wingate supramaximal test (WST) used with a purpose to reach a higher intensity in exercise matched with a short duration. The index of performance was defined in a software (WINGATE TEST®, CEFISE, BRASIL) to determine the power by each second during the test, beyond the relative peak power (RPP) (W.kg⁻¹), relative mean power (RMP) (W.kg⁻¹), fatigue index (FI) (%) and the peak power instant (PPI). The figure 9 represents the second study protocol.

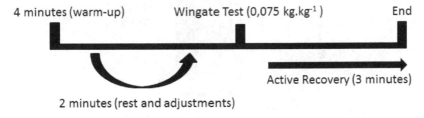

**Figure 9.** Illustrative representation of second study protocol, involving burst analyze.

The protocol consisted of 4 minutes warm-up in a mechanic cycle ergometer to lower limbs (MONARK 324E, SWEDEN) with 50 W load, with a pedal cadence in 70 rpm and the beginning of each minute the subjects realized a sprint during 6 seconds. After warm-up, the subjects rest for two minutes and they began the test, with a 0,075 kg.kg⁻¹ load until finish the test in 30 seconds. The same muscles were analyzed with the same EMG protocol and the same equipment's and procedures in the previous study. However, for this study in addition to the RMS also analyzed spectral parameters. To spectral analyses or frequency domain, was obtained the parameters from median frequency (MF), variance and slope, those values were determined using Wavelet Daubechies db4 (DWT) [6,8]. Was considered the analyses of EMG signal in the contraction phase (bursts) and during all signal (bursts + silence).

The table 2 present a descriptive analyze referent of subject performance.

| Variables | Men<br>n=14 | Women<br>n=13 |
|---|---|---|
| RPP (W.kg⁻¹) | 10.0 ± 0.9 | 7.7 ± 0,9 |
| RMP (W.kg⁻¹) | 7.3 ± 0.5 | 5.6 ± 0.6 |
| FI (%) | 52.9 ± 9,0 | 51.1 ± 11.9 |

Note: relative peak power (RPP), relative mean power (RMP), and fatigue index (FI).

**Table 2.** Mean values ± standard deviation of subject performance.

# 4. Results

## 4.1. Influence of the treatments (First study)

The figure 10 shows a comparative analyses of the RMS mean values from quadriceps integrated, obtained in submaximal intensity. We can see that no differences were found among different kinds of EMG treatment ($p > 0.05$), although it shows a tendency to decrease the values encountered in the measure that the procedure of analyses are added to treatment.

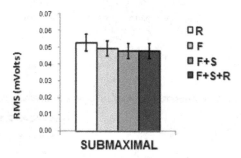

**Figure 10.** RMS values (mean and standard deviation) from quadriceps integrated muscles ([VL + VM+ RF] ÷ 3) in the different kinds of treatments to submaximal intensity exercise. R = Raw, F = Filtered, S = Smoothing. No differences were found ($p > 0.05$).

The figure 11 shows a comparative analyses of the RMS mean values from quadriceps integrated, obtained in maximal intensity. We can see that no differences were found among different kinds of EMG treatment ($p > 0.05$), although, like the submaximal intensity, it shows a tendency to decrease the values encountered in the measure that the procedure of analyses are added to treatment.

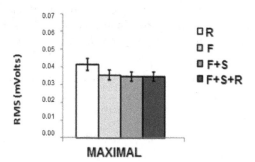

**Figure 11.** RMS values (mean and standard deviation) from quadriceps integrated muscles ([VL + VM+ RF] ÷ 3) in the different kinds of treatments to maximal intensity exercise. R = Raw, F = Filtered, S = Smoothing. No differences were found ($p > 0.05$).

The figure 12 shows a comparative analyses of the RMS mean values from quadriceps integrated, obtained in supramaximal intensity. Once again we can see that no differences were found among different kinds of EMG treatment (p>0.05), although, like the other two intensities, it shows a tendency to decrease the values encountered in the measure that the procedure of analyses are added to treatment.

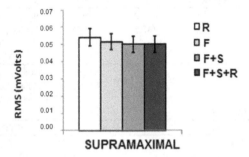

**Figure 12.** RMS values (mean and standard deviation) from quadriceps integrated muscles ([VL + VM+ RF] ÷ 3) in the different kinds of treatments to supramaximal intensity exercise. R = Raw, F = Filtered, S = Smoothing. No differences were found (p>0.05).

This last one is the one that most called our attention, once that an exercise in this intensity should cause a lot of noises, coming from the exercise (Cross-talk, muscular and skin movement, changes in the conductor tissues) and from the devices (electrode, wire movement, quickly distance change from the devices that capture and record the signal).

The Bland-Altman test shows good concordance between different methods of treatment in the neuromuscular activity to obtain the RMS in all muscles. In submaximal, maximal or supramaximal intensity differences among data weren`t found using as reference always the FSR method.

In trying to find possible influences of the EMG treatments procedures for the RMS value, the results allow us through the comparison and concordance tested to affirm a similar achievement in mVolts, for the muscles in any intensity. Those results shall bring us some perspective about the protocol imposed, where the principal recommendations are the filtering, rectification and smoothing [11]. The final results founded for the treatment of the muscular activity has a identification with a specific baseline achievement always close to zero [15]. Thus, the EMG is a very detailed and disturbed situation because of the sequence of noises, often caused by different reasons of difficulty control. It is worth to say the cross-talk influence, defined by the capitation of electric signal from synergic muscles. This interference normally doesn't surpass 15% of the total signal, but make it very clear the importance of a good location for the electrode. Also, a lot of different reasons can bring those noises, like the pressure, the environment and even the evaluator experience [16,18-20]. Thus, it's clear the necessities of procedures that can eliminate those noises, and give us a signal that really represents the muscular activity.

| SUBMAXIMAL (n=20) | | | BLAND and ALTMAN TEST(μVolt) | | | |
|---|---|---|---|---|---|---|
| TREATMENTS | | | ICC | BIAS | LD | UD |
| RF FRS | and | RF R | 0.927 | -0.0030 | -0.0120 | 0.0060 |
| RF FRS | and | RF F | 1.000 | -0.0002 | -0.0010 | 0.0006 |
| RF FRS | and | RF FS | 1.000 | 0.0000 | 0.0000 | 0.0000 |
| TREATMENTS RF | | | 0.980 | -------- | -------- | -------- |
| VM_FRS | and | VM_R | 0.958 | -0.0058 | -0.0275 | 0.0154 |
| VM FRS | and | VM F | 1.000 | -0.0008 | -0.0023 | 0.0008 |
| VM FRS | and | VM FS | 1.000 | 0.0000 | 0.0000 | 0.0000 |
| TREATMENTS VM | | | 0.989 | -------- | -------- | -------- |
| VL FRS | and | VL R | 0.830 | -0.0050 | -0.0247 | 0.0143 |
| VL FRS | and | VL F | 0.999 | -0.0008 | -0.0023 | 0.0008 |
| VL FRS | and | VL FS | 1.000 | 0.0000 | 0.0000 | 0.0000 |
| TREATMENTS VL | | | 0.959 | -------- | -------- | -------- |
| MAXIMAL (n=20) | | | BLAND and ALTMAN TEST (μVolt) | | | |
| TREATMENTS | | | ICC | BIAS | LD | UD |
| RF FRS | and | RF R | 0.950 | -0.0038 | -0.0151 | 0.0074 |
| RF FRS | and | RF F | 1.000 | -0.0006 | -0.0018 | 0.0006 |
| RF FRS | and | RF FS | 1.000 | 0.0000 | 0.0000 | 0.0000 |
| TREATMENTS RF | | | 0.987 | -------- | -------- | -------- |
| VM FRS | and | VM R | 0.994 | -0.0039 | -0.0075 | -0.0004 |
| VM FRS | and | VM F | 0.998 | -0.0022 | -0.0047 | 0.0003 |
| VM FRS | and | VM FS | 1.000 | 0.0000 | 0.0000 | 0.0000 |
| TREATMENTS VM | | | 0,999 | -------- | -------- | -------- |
| VL FRS | and | VL R | 0.969 | -0.0070 | -0.0209 | 0.0067 |
| VL FRS | and | VL F | 0.999 | -0.0015 | -0.0032 | 0.0003 |
| VL FRS | and | VL FS | 1.000 | 0.0000 | 0.0000 | 0.0000 |
| TREATMENTS VL | | | 0.992 | -------- | -------- | -------- |
| SUPRAMAXIMAL (n=20) | | | BLAND and ALTMAN TEST (μVolt) | | | |
| TREATMENTS | | | ICC | BIAS | LD | UD |
| RF FRS | and | RF R | 0.970 | -0.0022 | -0.0063 | 0.0019 |
| RF FRS | and | RF F | 0.999 | -0.0004 | -0.0016 | 0.0008 |
| RF FRS | and | RF FS | 1.000 | 0.0000 | 0.0000 | 0.0000 |
| TREATMENTS RF | | | 0.993 | -------- | -------- | -------- |
| VM FRS | and | VM R | 0.992 | -0.0048 | -0.0114 | 0.0016 |
| VM FRS | and | VM F | 0.999 | -0.0020 | -0.0042 | 0.0003 |
| VM FRS | and | VM FS | 1.000 | 0.0000 | 0.0000 | 0.0000 |
| TREATMENTS VM | | | 0.998 | -------- | -------- | -------- |
| VL FRS | and | VL R | 0.992 | -0.0039 | -0.0087 | 0.0009 |
| VL FRS | and | VL F | 0.999 | -0.0018 | -0.0040 | 0.0004 |
| VL FRS | and | VL FS | 1.000 | 0.0000 | 0.0000 | 0.0000 |
| TREATMENTS VL | | | 0.998 | -------- | -------- | -------- |

RF: Rectu Femoris; VM: Vastus Medialis; VL: Vastus Lateralis; FRS: Filtered, Rectified, Smooth; R: Raw; F: Filtered; FS: Filtered, Smooth.

**Table 3.** Intraclass Correlation Coefficient (ICC), Bias Level of treatment (BIAS) and Lower Dispersion (LD) Upper Dispersion (UD) from BIAS in submaximal, maximal and supramaximal exercise.

## 4.2. Influence of the burst and silence in treatment of EMG signal (Second Study)

The figure 13 present us the RMS comparison between different kinds of analyze (all signal phase and contraction phase) respectively, among muscles: RF, VM and VL in the Wingate Test, no differences were found between methods (p>0.05).

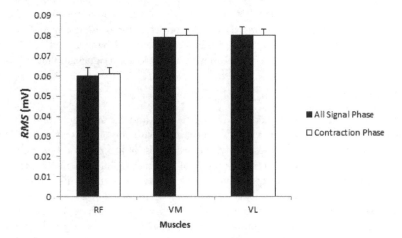

**Figure 13.** Comparison of root mean square (RMS) between three different muscles from quadriceps femoris (RF = rectus femoris, VM = vastus lateralis, VL = vastus lateralis) in a Wingate Test (p>0.05).

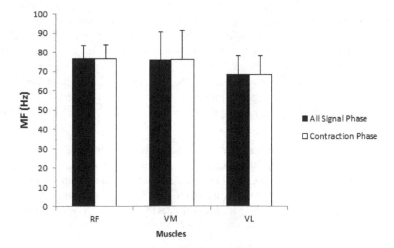

**Figure 14.** Comparison of Median Frequency (MF) between three different muscles from quadriceps femoris (RF = rectus femoris, VM = vastus lateralis, VL = vastus lateralis) in a Wingate Test (p>0.05).

The figure 14 present us the MF comparison between different kinds of analyze (all signal phase and contraction phase) respectively, among muscles: RF, VM and VL in the Wingate test, no differences were found between methods (p>0.05).

The results presented above show us that there were no significant difference between the two analyzes. Probably, these results were found because despite the silence moment has power gradient, the amount of lost energy is not enough to change the EMG signal parameters when the whole signal is analyzed. This result should not be transferred to others activity like the golf or to a martial art kick or punch for example due to the different characteristics, where in this sports the motor activity should be analyzed per complete, because during the whole time there is a contraction, so there is a signal amplitude [21-22].

## 5. Conclusions

We concluded that, although exist many orientations and recommendations to use and apply the electromyography method, sometimes these components can be a path too complex to understand and to respect with closed eyes. In a considerable perspective of study we were able to show with a model of exercise in high intensity, which was capable to produce a lot of noises and variations on the signal, that different methods of process to achieve the muscular activity do not change the final result if used the complete signal or just the burst parts, or still using all sequence of treatment with filtration, rectification and smoothing in many combinations of analyses. Moreover, should be noted that only filtration was sufficient to improve the quality of EMG signal, making us think in keeping the use at least the filtration in electromyography analyses, still this procedure is used to at least maintain the signal inside the muscle activity range, so, it should not be took out just because no significant differences were founded, we have to consider all the process, as said before, like the devices used and the investigator experience. These outcomes show us that we have remained with a critical knowledge to many things and test the main recommendations to use some techniques. In order to make those results clearer and give us more confidence when use the treatments in EMG analyzes. Some studies creating different noises in computer should be made. This way we can be more secure about the removing of noises, securing that the absence of difference is not because a good pre-acquisition was made, securing not enough noises to be cut.

These results and conclusion takes in consideration only cyclic exercise with the intensity used in the studies. Exercises such as isometric or acyclic have different signal waves and so, could have different results to the same treatments. Also, exercises with lower load could change mainly the results in the Burst + Silence (Second Study) results, once that a task such as 10 km in low intensity, would be realized with less intense movements, creating not only different power signals but also different silence and burst time duration.

Still, a more accuracy statistic method could be used, such as The Smallest Worthwhile Change [23], capable to find minimal and almost invisible differences between different methods, that can contribute with good perspective to sports domain when obscure changes exist among several techniques to data process in EMG analysis and if we use a classical statistic we may not identify with probabilities these modulations.

## 6. Future directions

Although, we should now take the conclusions and think in considerable applicability with our outcomes, we should remain our critical thinking about the theme, about our limitations and keep our considerations related just to our results in this study with these methods and these subjects. We expect that our findings encourage new experiences inside a positive vision in his complete trend to refute ours dogmas and explain in a better way how we should use and respect the recommendations and orientations to electromyography application in human studies, involving different kind of exercise in several intensities and oscillating between isometric and isotonic conditions, testing many aspects that stays around electromyography process and show to the scientific world a great amount of specificities to use this technique taking into account these variables capable to confuse and change the signal with noises, underestimating or overestimating the final value.

Such design, as showed on this chapter should be applied to others tasks with the same characteristics, like running or any other cyclic exercises that has different muscles involved with different activation ranges and other kinds of possible noises, and silence and burst times. Also, different data process should be tested for spectral analyses, like Wavelet families and Fast Fourier Transform (FFT) for different exercises modalities, until it comes to conclusion about the correct use of this technique involving the correct results achievement, signal process and interpretation.

## 7. Nomenclature

EMG – Electromyography
RMS – Root Mean Square
MIT – Maximal Incremental Test
MWL – Maximal Work Load
CLT – Constant Load Test
Rpm – Revolution per Minute
ISEK - International Society of Electrophysiology and Kinesiology
SENIAM – Surface Electromyography for Non-Invasive Assessment of Muscles
R- Raw signal
F – Filtrated Signal
FS – Filtrated and Smoothed signal
FSR – Signal Filtrated, Smoothed and Rectified
RF – Rectus Femoris
VM – Vastus Medialis
VL – Vastus Lateralis
ICC – Interclass Correlation Coefficient
BIAS – Bias Level of Treatment

LD – Lower Dispersion from BIAS
UD – Upper Dispersion from BIAS
FI – Fatigue Index
PPI – Peak Power Instant
MF – Median
RPP – Relative Peak Power
RMP – Relative Mean Power

## Author details

Leandro Ricardo Altimari, José Luiz Dantas,
Marcelo Bigliassi and Thiago Ferreira Dias Kanthack
*Group of Study and Research in Neuromuscular System and Exercise,*
*CEFE - State University of Londrina, Brazil*

Antonio Carlos de Moraes
*GPNeurom - Laboratory of Electromyography Studies, FEF - State University of Campinas, Brazil*

Taufik Abrão
*Department of Electrical Engineering, CTU - State University of Londrina, Brazil*

## Acknowledgement

We are thankful to everyone of the Laboratory of Telecomunications and DSP (Department of Electrical Engineering/CTU, State University of Londrina) and to Dra. Maria Angelica O. C. Brunetto (Department of Computing/CCE, State University of Londrina) that helped with the development of MatLab routine to process the electromyography data and give us the possibility to understand in different perspectives the same cue. The authors thank still the Fundação Araucária do Paraná, the Fundação de Amparo a Pesquisa do Estado de São Paulo (FAPESP), and Conselho Nacional de Desenvolvimento Cientifico e Tecnológico (CNPq) for post-graduate scholarships and supported financially. Finally we say thanks to everybody that meticulously contributed with this work, in your write or review process, and additionally keep in thankful to professor Dr. Ganesh Naik for given us the possibility to be part of this wonderful work, helping others to understand the electromyography in cyclic activities.

## 8. References

[1] Medved, V. & Cifrek, M. Kinesiological electromyography. Biomechanics in applications.4(7) 2010; 349-366.

[2] Massó, N., Rey, F., Romero, D., GuaL, G., Ccosta, L. & Germám, A. Surface electromyography applications in the sport. Apunts Medicina del I'Esport. 2010;45(165) 121-130.

[3] Camata, T. V., AltimarI, L. R., Bortolotti, H., Dantas, J. L. et al. Electromyographic Activity and Rate of Muscle Fatigue of the Quadriceps Femoris During Cycling Exercise

in the Severe Domain. Journal Strength and Conditioning Research.2011;25(9) 2537-2543.

[4] Andrade, M. M., nascimento, F. A. O. Análise tempo-frequência de sinais eletromiográficos de superfície para a avaliação de fadiga muscular em cicloergômetro. Tese de doutorado, UNB. Brasília. 2006.

[5] Ocarino, J. M., Silva, P. L. P., Vaz, D. V., Aquino, C. F., Brício, R. S., Fonseca, S. T. Eletromiografia: interpretação e aplicações nas ciências da reabilitação. Fisioterapia. Brasil. 2005;6(4) 305-310.

[6] Dantas, J. L., Camata, T. V., Brunetto, M. A. O. C., Moraes, A. C., Abrao, T., Altimari, L. R. Fourier (STFT) and Wavelet (db4) spectral analysis of EMG signals in isometric and dynamic maximal effort exercise. IEEE Engineering in Medicine and Biology Society. Conf. 2010:1(1) 5979-5982.

[7] Vitor-Costa, M., Pereira, L. A., Oliveria, R. S., Pedro, R. E., Camata, T. V., Abrao, T., Brunetto, M. A. O. C.,Altimari, L. R. Fourier (STFT) and Wavelet (db4) spectral analysis of EMG signals in maximal cosntant load dynamic exercise. IEEE Engineering in Medicine and Biology Society. Conf. 2010 : 1(1) 4622-4625.

[8] Camata, T. V., Dantas, J. L., Abrao, T., Brunetto, M. A. O. C., Moraes, A. C., Altimari, L. R. Fourier (STFT) and Wavelet (db4) spectral analysis of EMG signals in supramaximal constant load dymic exercise. IEEE Engineering in Medicine and Biology Society. Conf. 2010: 1(1) 1364 - 1367.

[9] Kamen, G. & Gabriell, D. A. Essentials of electromyography. Champaign, IL: Human Kinetics. 2010.

[10] Farina, D. Interpretation of the surface electromyogram in dynamic contractions. Exercise and Sports Science Review; 2006(34)3 121-7.

[11] Konrad, P. The ABC of EMG: A Practical Introduction to Kinesiological Electromyography. Version 1.0 April, Noraxon INC. USA. 2005

[12] Hermens, H, J., Freriks, B., Disselhorst-klug, C. & Rau, G. Development of recommendations for SEMG sensors and sensor placement procedures. Journal of Electromyography and Kinesiology. 2000;10(5) 361-374.

[13] Pezarat, C. P. & Santos, P. A Electromiografia no Estudo do Movimento Humana. Faculdade de Motricidade Humana. Lisboa. 2004.

[14] Camata, T. V., et al. Association between the electromyographic fatigue threshold and ventilatory threshold. Electromyography and Clinical Neurophysiology. 2009;49(6-7) 102-108.

[15] De luca, C. J., Gilmore, L. D., Kuznetsov, M. & Roy, S. R. Filtering the surface EMG signal: Movement artifact and baseline noise contamination. Journal of Biomechanics. 2010;43 (8) 1573-9

[16] Merletti, R., et al. Surface electromyography for noninvasive characterization of muscle. Exercise and Sports Sciences Reviews. 2001;29(1) 20-25.

[17] Finsterer, J. EMG-interference pattern analysis. Journal of Electromyography and Kinesiology.2011;11(4) 231-46.

[18] Clancy, E. A., Morin, E. L. & Merletti, R. Sampling, noise-reduction and amplitude estimation issues in surface electromyography. Journal of Electromyography and Kinesiology. 2002;1(12) 1-16.

[19] Mclean, L., Chislett, M., Murphy, M. & Walton, P. The effect of head position, electrode site, movement and smoothing window in the determination of a reliable maximum voluntary activation of the upper trapezius muscle. Journal of Electromyography and Kinesiology. 2003;2(13) 169–180.

[20] Disselhorst-klug, C., Schmitz-rode, T. & Rau, G. Surface electromyography and muscle force: Limits in sEMG–force relationship and new approaches for applications. Clinical Biomechanics. 2009;3(24) 225-235.

[21] Vencesbrito, A. M. et al. Kinematic and electromyographic analyses of a karate punch. Journal of Electromyography and Kinesiology. 2011; 21(6) 1023-1029.

[22] Farber, A. J. et al. Electromyographic analysis of forearm muscles in professional and amateur golfers. American Journal of Sports Medicine. 2009;37(2) 396-401.

[23] Hopkins, W. G., et al. Progressive statistics for studies in sports medicine and exercise science. Medicine and Science in Sports and Exercise. 2009; 41(1) 3-13.

# EMG Applications:
# Hand Gestures and Prosthetics

# Chapter 6

# Hand Sign Classification Employing Myoelectric Signals of Forearm

Takeshi Tsujimura, Sho Yamamoto and Kiyotaka Izumi

Additional information is available at the end of the chapter

## 1. Introduction

Electromyogram (EMG) signals are generated in muscles, when the muscles contract and a joint is flexed or extended. EMG signals can be measured from a skin surface with noninvasive electrodes, and they include some information on motions such as muscle torque or joint angles. Hence, it is possible to achieve more intuitive human-machine interface using EMG signals than conventional interfaces such as joysticks, data gloves, motion captures. Various interfaces using EMG signals have been proposed to control robot hands (Graupe et al.; Jacobson et al.; Yoshikawa et al., 2009; Ibe at al.). Some methods for hand motion identification have been reported since the 1990s based on soft-computing approaches, e. g. artificial neural networks (Fukuda et al.; Hudgins et al.), fuzzy logic (Karlik & Tokhi; Chan et al.), support vector machine (Yoshikawa et al., 2007; Oskoei & Huosheng), and so on (Chen et al.; Huang et al.). These approaches have improved accuracy of motion discrimination and the number of discriminated motions. However, they need complicated processes and huge amount of calculations.

The purpose of our study is to design an uncomplicated system to identify finger motion and to develop innovative human-machine interfaces. We began with the investigation of the forearm muscle EMG (Tsujimura et al.; Yamamoto et al.). We supposed that not only finger muscles but forearm ones work when the knuckles display hand signs. For this purpose, an EMG measurement system is constructed first to detect surface EMG signals of a forearm and to convert them to more manageable types of features. We next evaluate the correlation between the forearm EMG signals and finger motions. It discloses the activity pattern of each forearm muscle corresponding to specific hand sign. The identification algorithm of hand signs is then designed based on the optimized criterion of muscle activity. Finally, identification of finger gesture is experimented to demonstrate the effectiveness of our proposed method.

## 2. EMG measurement system

### 2.1. Measurement system design

Block diagram of our EMG measurement system is shown in Fig. 1. Surface EMG signals are measured with three electrodes placed on a forearm. The EMG signals are preprocessed and converted into integrated EMG (IEMG) signals through the EMG measurement instrument. An IEMG signal has been used as an index of a muscle activity level in exercise physiology (Milner-Brown & Stein). Both EMG and IEMG are introduced into a PC to evaluate the averaged IEMG (AIEMG) features. An estimation algorithm of finger gesture is installed in the PC. After determining criterions of muscle activity, the proposed system identifies motions of fingers.

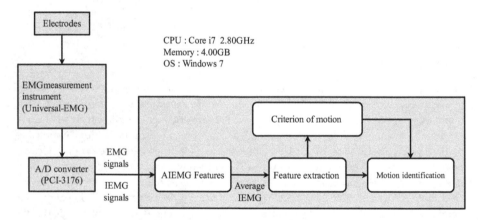

**Figure 1.** EMG measurement system

Figure 2 illustrates the forearm muscles whose EMG signals are measured by the instrument, and the positions of three electrodes placed on the forearm. The center figure shows forearm cross section of anatomical muscle placement.

Extensor pollicis brevis monitored with the electrode 1 (channel 1) is involved in finger extension. Extensor digitorum monitored with the electrode 2 (channel 2) is also involved in finger extension. Flexor digitorum profundus monitored with the electrode 3 (channel 3) is involved in finger flexion.

The EMG signals are measured with bipolar surface electrodes consisting of two parallel silver bars. These signals are amplified and converted into IEMG signals with rectification smoothing (the cutoff frequency 2.4 Hz) by means of a differential amplifier (Universal-EMG, Oisaka development Ltd.). The EMG signals are sampled at 10 kHz through a 16-bit A/D converter (PCI-3176, Interface Co.) and taken in a data-collection computer (Core i7 2.8 GHz, Windows 7).

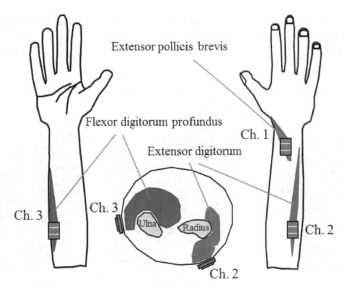

**Figure 2.** Measured muscles and electrodes placed on forearm

## 2.2. Electromyogram features

The AIEMG feature is a periodic average of EMG signals during a designated interval (Yoshikawa et al., 2007). It is extracted from the IEMG in the 100 ms frame, which is shifted for 12.5 ms (80 Hz). Hamming window functions are applied to the signals in each frame. Since the measured data is converted into digital quantity by the PC interface, the AIEMG is calculated in terms of the moving average of the IEMG magnitude as

$$AIEMG(k) = \frac{1}{N} \sum_{t=0}^{N-1} IEMG(t), \, , \tag{1}$$

where AIEMG(k), and IEMG(t) represent the AIEMG feature of the k-th averaging frame and the IEMG magnitude of the t-th sample within the frame, respectively. Number of samples in a frame is denoted by N.

The AIEMG eliminates momentary noise such as a spike, because it is a kind of low-pass filters. The larger you take the sampling number, the smoother the AIEMG signal becomes. If you choose N=1, the AIEMG is the same as the IEMG signal.

## 3. Forearm EMG signals regarding finger motion

Not only muscles of fingers but of forearms work when you use your fingers. First of all, we have investigated the relationship between finger motion and the forearm EMG signals. Although we have obtained fundamental responses with regard to each single finger motion, this paper focuses only on typical gestures of composite finger configurations.

"Rock-paper-scissors" is a hand game played by two or more people. Each player changes his hand into one of three basic hand-signs representing rock, paper, or scissors as shown in Fig. 3. Each of the hand signs beats one of the other two, and loses to the other in the game.

Our purpose in this paper is to distinguish the hand-signs by analyzing the forearm EMG signals.

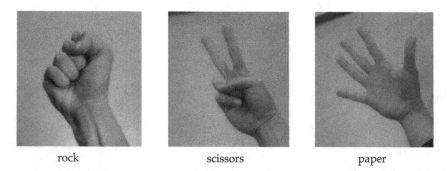

|            rock            |           scissors           |            paper            |

**Figure 3.** Hand signs to be distinguished

## 3.1. EMG and IEMG signals

We have evaluated the forearm EMG signals with our measurement system. When displaying "rock" by clenching fist, the EMG and IEMG signals were measured as shown in Figs. 4 and 5. Figure 4 (a1), (a2), and (a3) indicate the EMG signals measured with channels 1, 2, and 3, respectively, where the horizontal axis expresses time, and the vertical represents magnitude of the EMG signal. The IEMG signals are also evaluated as shown in Fig. 5. Figure 5 (b1), (b2), and (b3) indicate the IEMG signals measured with channels 1, 2, and 3, respectively, where the horizontal axis expresses time and the vertical represents magnitude of the IEMG signal. Those waveforms shown in Figs. 4 and 5 indicate that channel 1 is inactive, channel 2 is less active, and only channel 3 is active. It can be considered that flexor digitorum profundus is mainly working when you shape "rock" with your hand.

"Scissors" are represented by two fingers extended and separated. The EMG and IEMG signals were measured regarding "scissors" as shown in Figs. 6 and 7, respectively. These figures show that channel 2 is solely active and channels 1 and 3 are almost inactive. Results support that extensor digitorum contributes to showing "scissors."

An open hand signifies "paper." The EMG and IEMG signals are shown with regard to "paper" in Figs. 8 and 9, respectively. They indicate both channels 1 and 2 are active and channel 3 is less active. It is surmised that "paper" is formed owing to both extensor pollicis brevis and extensor digitorum.

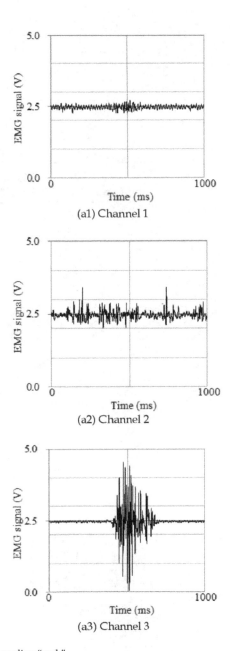

**Figure 4.** EMG signals regarding "rock"

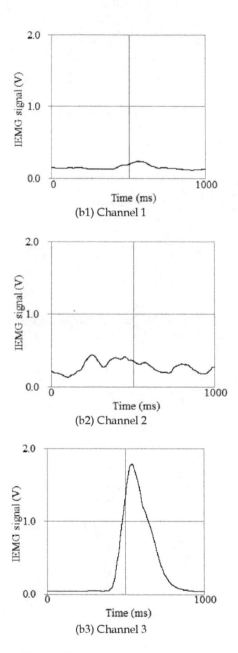

**Figure 5.** IEMG signals regarding "rock"

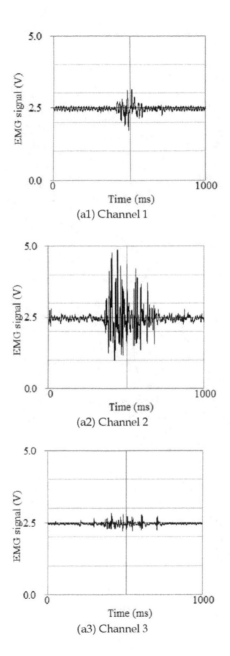

**Figure 6.** EMG signals regarding "scissors"

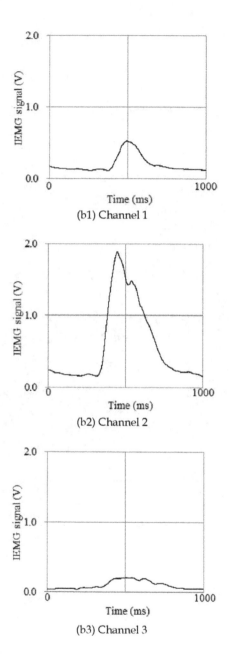

**Figure 7.** IEMG signals regarding "scissors"

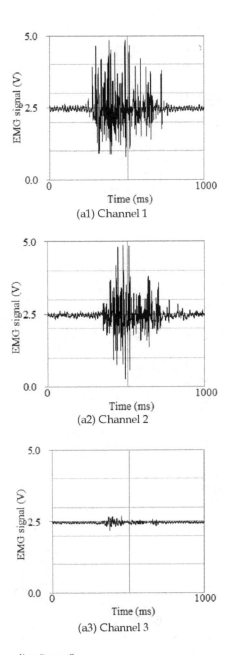

**Figure 8.** EMG signals regarding "paper"

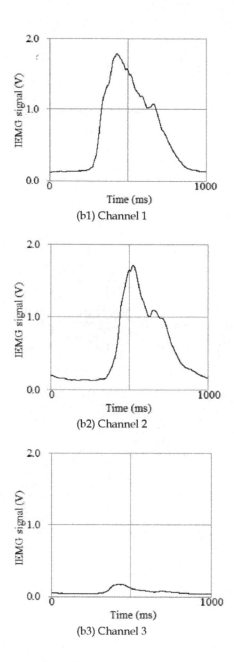

**Figure 9.** IEMG signals regarding "paper"

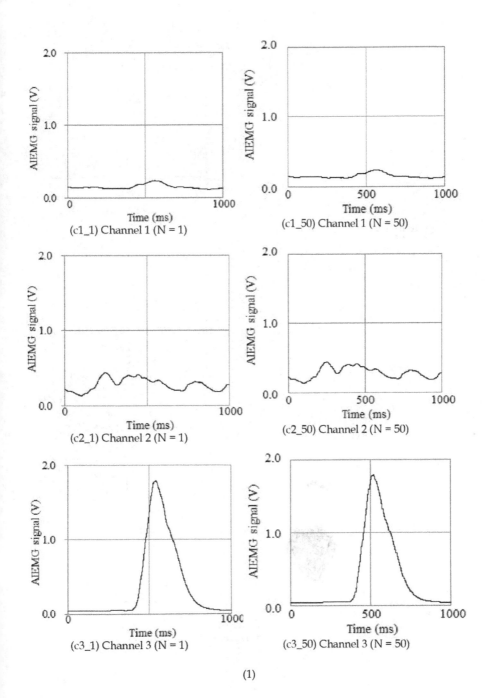

(c1_1) Channel 1 (N = 1)

(c1_50) Channel 1 (N = 50)

(c2_1) Channel 2 (N = 1)

(c2_50) Channel 2 (N = 50)

(c3_1) Channel 3 (N = 1)

(c3_50) Channel 3 (N = 50)

(1)

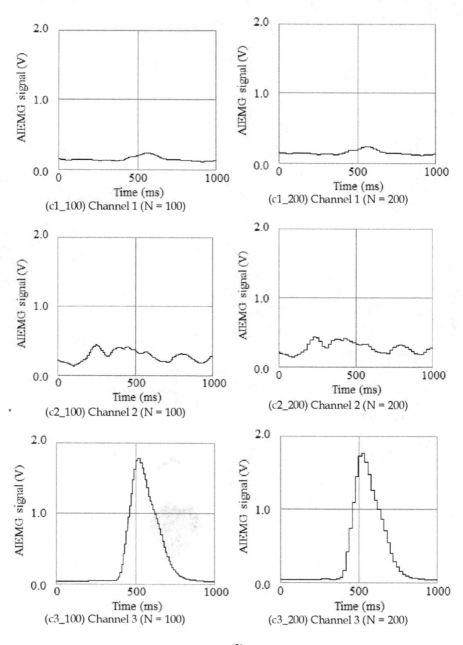

(c1_100) Channel 1 (N = 100)

(c1_200) Channel 1 (N = 200)

(c2_100) Channel 2 (N = 100)

(c2_200) Channel 2 (N = 200)

(c3_100) Channel 3 (N = 100)

(c3_200) Channel 3 (N = 200)

(2)

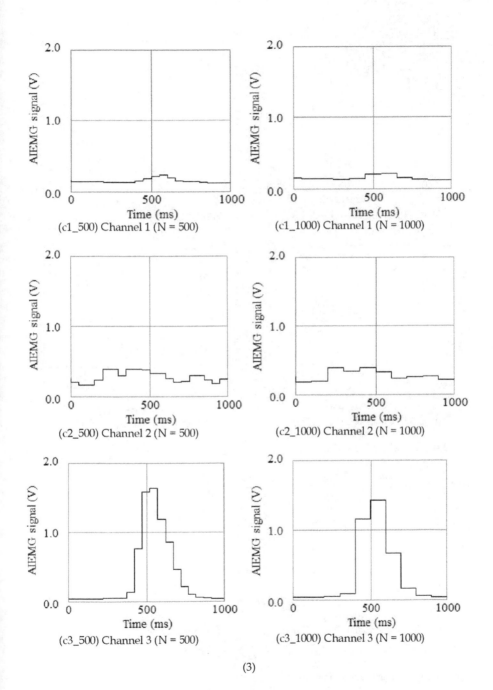

(c1_500) Channel 1 (N = 500)

(c1_1000) Channel 1 (N = 1000)

(c2_500) Channel 2 (N = 500)

(c2_1000) Channel 2 (N = 1000)

(c3_500) Channel 3 (N = 500)

(c3_1000) Channel 3 (N = 1000)

(3)

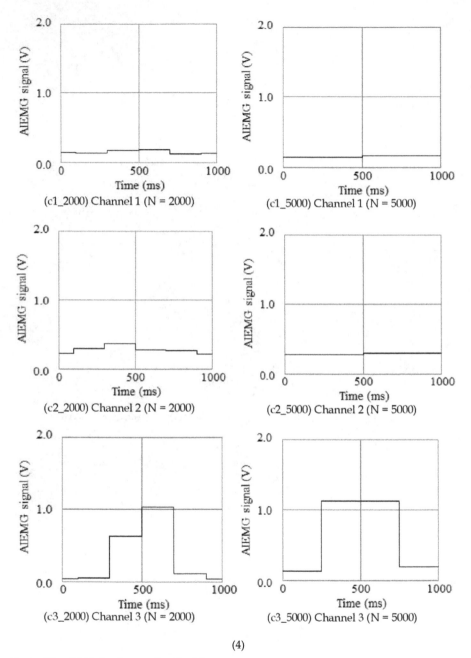

(4)

**Figure 10.** AIEMG signals regarding "rock"

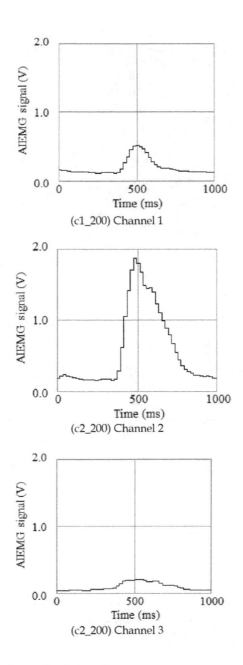

(N = 200)

**Figure 11.** AIEMG signals regarding "scissors"

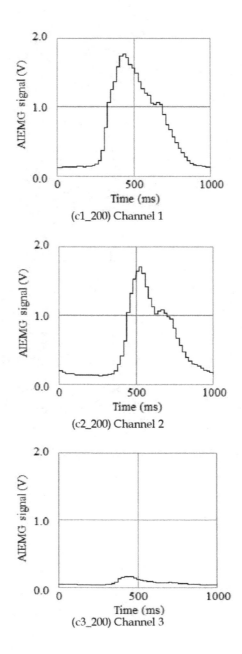

(c1_200) Channel 1

(c2_200) Channel 2

(c3_200) Channel 3

(N = 200)

**Figure 12.** AIEMG signals regarding "paper"

## 3.2. AIEMG signals

We next calculated the averaged IEMG (AIEMG) signals from IEMG according to eq. (1). They are stable and noiseless compared to the IEMG, because the feature prevents instantaneous noise of IEMG signals. It is important to adopt the optimum sampling number, N, to obtain the ideal AIEMG feature. When the number is too small, the signal intensity fluctuates and it is difficult to obtain consistent feature at every measurement. If it is too large, the AIEMG signal becomes blunt and thus its original waveform is lost.

Figure 10 shows the examples of AIEMG derived from IEMG signals indicated in Fig. 5, with regard to the number of sampling, N as 1, 50, 100, 200, 500, 1000, 2000, and 5000.

Figure 10(c1_1), for instance, displays the AIEMG signal measured by channels 1 with sampling number of 1, where the horizontal axis expresses time, and the vertical represents magnitude of the AIEMG signal.

Figures 11 and 12 are representations of the AIEMG signals regarding channels 2 and 3, respectively, whose sampling number is 200.

## 4. Finger sign identification based on forearm AIEMG signals

### 4.1. Muscle activity corresponding to finger sign

When evaluating the experimental results, we have Table 1 which indicates contribution of muscles to gesticulation by hands. Extensor pollicis brevis does its part only in displaying "paper" among three signs. Extensor digitorum works when forming "scissors" and "paper." Flexor digitorum profundus contributes only to indication of "rock."

This table helps us to classify displayed finger signs based only on the forearm surface EMG signals in real time. If obtaining any of the specific EMG signal combinations shown in the table, we can deduce one of the finger signs among three.

Note that an electrode does not necessarily catch signals only when the corresponding muscle works. Thus, it is necessary to differentiate active signals from inactive to identify muscle motion precisely.

| Muscle | | Rock | Scissors | Paper |
|---|---|---|---|---|
| Ch.1 | Extensor pollicis brevis | × | × | ○ |
| Ch.2 | Extensor digitorum | × | ○ | ○ |
| Ch.3 | Flexor digitorum profundus | ○ | × | × |

○: Active ×: Inactive

**Table 1.** Muscle activity pattern for finger sign

### 4.2. Criterion of muscle activity

We have next investigated an identification of finger signs by analyzing the AIEMG of a forearm. The EMG signals were detected by three electrodes put on the forearm skin of the subjects, and active signals were distinguished from inactive ones according to the following principle. An algorithm for identifying finger motion was designed to refer the active/inactive combination described above.

We have measured the forearm EMG signals in advance to determine the criterion for each muscle to discriminate between active and inactive signals. The criteria were separately settled with regard to several sampling numbers by observing activity of the muscles. The activity is evaluated by the peak voltage of each AIEMG signal.

Ten trials were conducted by gesturing each of the hand shapes for each sampling number.

Experimental results are arranged in Fig. 13.

Figure 13(d1_1), for example, indicates the magnitude of 30 AIEMG waveforms detected by channel 1 with the sampling number of 1. The vertical axis represents the peak voltage of the AIEMG signal when the subject made gestures of "rock," "scissors," and "paper." It implys the activity of extensor pollicis brevis. We determined the criterion index, $CI_1$ for channel 1 at N=1 as 0.58 V, which is illustrated by a bold line in the figure.

The activity of muscles can be estimated according to the criteria as follows. Provided that the magnitude of a measured signal is larger than the criterion, the corresponding muscle is presumed to be active. Otherwise it is considered to be inactive.

All the data regarding "rock" and "scissors" were smaller than the line, while those for "paper" were larger in this figure. That is why we could surmise that extensor pollicis brevis is active only for "paper."

In the same way, the output AIEMG signals of channels 2 and 3 are arranged as for N=1 in Figs. 11 (d2_1) and (d3_1), respectively. The criterion indices, $CI_2$ and $CI_3$ for channel 2 and 3 were determined as 0.76 and 0.61 V, respectively. By acquired AIEMG signals of extensor digitorum, channel 2 indicated the muscle is active for "scissors" and "paper." Channel 3, representing the activity of flexor digitorum profundus, confirmed that the muscle is active only in the case of "rock."

Note that these experimental data support the classification patterns of finger signs shown in Table 1.

With respect to other sampling numbers, similar features were observed as shown in Fig.11(d1_50) - (d3_5000). Their corresponding criteria were determined as shown in Table 2.

| N | $CI_1$ (V) | $CI_2$ (V) | $CI_3$ (V) |
|---|---|---|---|
| 1 | 0.58 | 0.76 | 0.61 |
| 50 | 0.54 | 0.76 | 0.58 |
| 100 | 0.53 | 0.76 | 0.58 |
| 200 | 0.53 | 0.76 | 0.59 |
| 500 | 0.48 | 0.73 | 0.56 |
| 1000 | 0.47 | 0.71 | 0.51 |
| 2000 | 0.38 | 0.54 | 0.33 |
| 5000 | 0.22 | 0.40 | 0.23 |

**Table 2.** Criterion of muscle activity

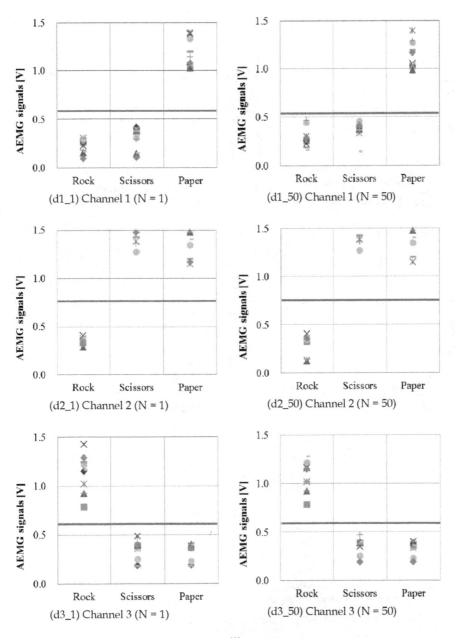

(d1_1) Channel 1 (N = 1)

(d1_50) Channel 1 (N = 50)

(d2_1) Channel 2 (N = 1)

(d2_50) Channel 2 (N = 50)

(d3_1) Channel 3 (N = 1)

(d3_50) Channel 3 (N = 50)

(1)

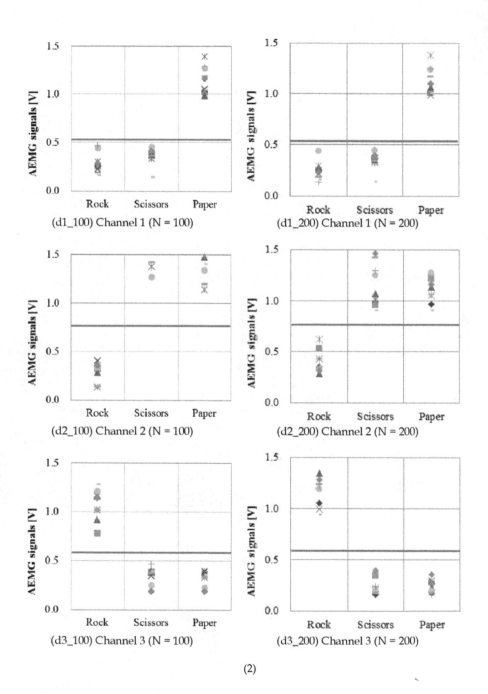

(2)

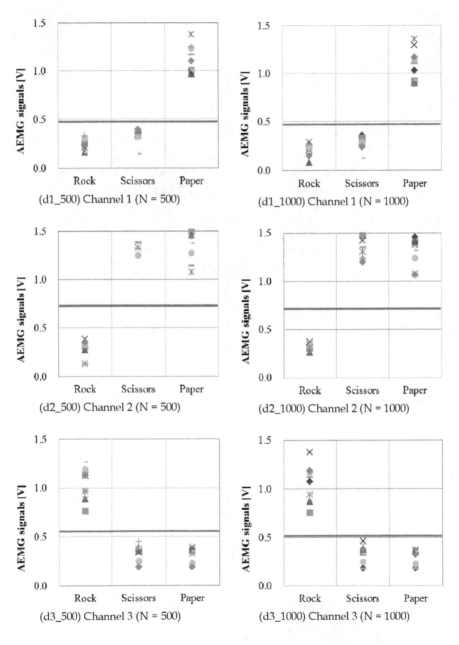

(3)

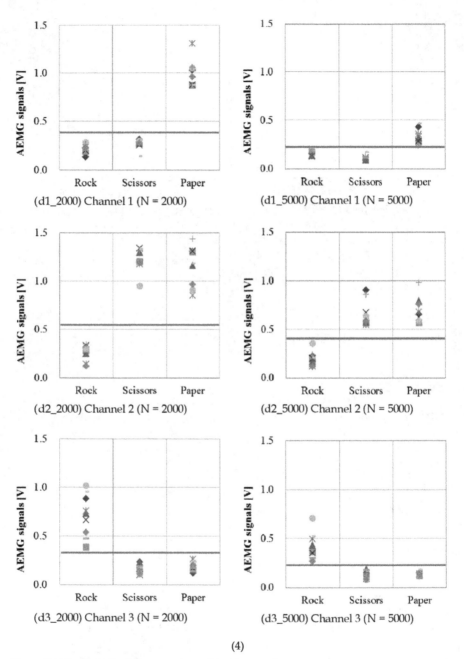

(4)

**Figure 13.** Discrimination between active and inactive muscle

## 4.3. Finger gesture estimation

A flowchart of the gesture estimation algorithm is shown in Fig. 14. First of all, the AIEMG features are calculated by eq. (1). Next, the peak intensity, $AIEMG_2$ of the AIEMG signal detected by channel 2 is compared with the criterion index, $CI_2$. Then, the intensities, $AIEMG_3$ and $AIEMG_1$ are weighed against the criterion indices, $CI_3$ and $CI_1$, respectively. This process checks the combination of the measured AIEMG signals against the activation patterns of muscles corresponding to the finger signs shown in Table 1.

We finally carried out the experiments of finger sign estimation based on the algorithm. Identification rate was evaluated after 40 trials were conducted for each finger sign. Several sampling numbers for AIEMG feature were investigated. Experimental results are indicated in Table 3 and Fig. 15, which show percentages of correct answers with regard to each sampling number. They suggest that N=200 is the optimum sampling number among our investigations after all. Detailed analysis clarified that larger sampling number, e. g. N=1000, deforms the signals into blunt waveforms and thus it occasionally prevents discriminating between active and inactive signals. On the other hand, the AIEMG signals contain some transient noise when the sampling number is too small. It caused misjudgment on discrimination of activity of extensor pollicis brevis, for instance, that is evaluated with electrode 1 (channel 1). It can be considered to be one of the reasons why the identification rate of "paper" is inferior to the others.

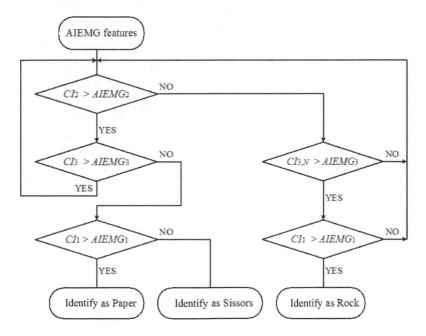

**Figure 14.** Finger sign estimation algorithm

| N | Rock (%) | Scissors (%) | Paper (%) | Total(%) |
|---|---|---|---|---|
| 1 | 97.5 | 87.5 | 57.5 | 80.8 |
| 50 | 97.5 | 97.5 | 65.0 | 86. 7 |
| 100 | 95.0 | 95.0 | 70.0 | 86. 7 |
| 200 | 97.5 | 97.5 | 97.5 | 97.5 |
| 500 | 95.0 | 85.0 | 70.0 | 83.3 |
| 1000 | 90.0 | 77.5 | 82.5 | 83.3 |
| 2000 | 80.0 | 62.5 | 57.5 | 66. 7 |
| 5000 | 37.5 | 27.5 | 20.0 | 28.3 |

**Table 3.** Accuracy rate of finger sign identification

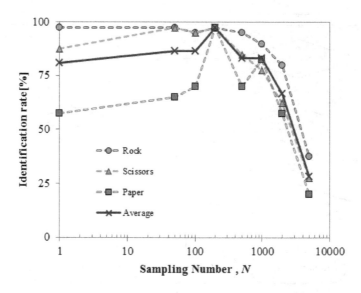

**Figure 15.** Experimental results of finger sign identification

## 5. Conclusion

We have studied the estimation method of hand signs employing the electromyogram. This paper focused on the forearm EMG signals caused by the finger motion. It relys on the proposition that the specific muscles of forearms work even if you only move your fingers.

First of all, the EMG measurement system was designed to detect signals from the surface skin of forearms. We constructed three-channel myoelectric signal processing system by assigning three forearm muscles; extensor pollicis brevis, extensor digitorum, and flexor digitorum profundus. It provided EMG and IEMG signals, and also calculated AIEMG features.

Fundamental experiments were carried out next to acquire data regarding the relationship between the finger motion and the forearm EMG signals. Investigation on myoelectric responses revealed that the specified forearm muscles were activated with respect to the corresponding finger motion.

The disclosed principles were applied to identification of typical hand signs such as "rock," "paper," and "scissors" in terms of the well-known hand game. We obtained correlative experimental data of hand signs and the myoelectric signals.

We found out the activity pattern of forearm muscles with regard to each hand sign as follows. If shaping "rock," flexor digitorum profundus is mainly working. When "scissors" are indicated, extensor digitorum is activated. Display of "paper" is owing to both extensor pollicis brevis and extensor digitorum.

We established the following principles in consequence to deduce the hand sign from the activities of forearm muscles. Extensor pollicis brevis is active in displaying "paper." Extensor digitorum operates when forming "scissors" and "paper." Flexor digitorum profundus contributes only to indication of "rock."

We then designed the classification algorithm based on the results. Because the myoelectric signals fluctuated and depended on the measurement conditions in reality, we determined the criterion of each muscle's activity by statistical treatment and we evaluated the averaged IEMG signals. The AIEMG functioned as a kind of low-pass filters, and its performance was dependent on the sampling number. We investigated the results of AIEMG features and determined the optimum sampling number was 200.

Finally, we conducted some experiments on real-time discrimination of three typical hand signs. The identification accuracy was no less than 97 % with respect to any hand sign when choosing the optimum sampling number.

Experimental results proved that the proper AIEMG feature was successful in inferring the shape of hands. We have confirmed the validity and effectiveness of our proposed estimation system at last. Thus, the method to estimate hand signs has been established based on the activity of forearm muscles instead of finger muscles.

## 6. Future directions

Our study was just started with myoelectrical analysis on the forearm muscles and finger motion. Proposed technique was applied to the hand game called "rock-paper-scissors." But it was configured so as to verify the validity of the method rather than to demonstrate its usefulness.

We are planning to improve the technique to human-robot interface system. The advanced input device for computers is one of the applications, which is more intuitive than the data-glove. Such versatile system is neccesary to distinguish many finger motions based on vague myoelectric information.

This paper evaluated the myoelectric signals processed simply by statistic evaluation for noise reduction or feature extraction. Higher performance may be expected by introducing some meta-heuristic method or intelligent method, e. g. neural networks, or suppot vector machine.

The muscle activity was determined on the basis of dualistic taxology according to the criterion established beforehand in this paper. It is necessary to determine the criterion adaptively to the measument conditions to apply to realtime robotic systems.

Practical systems will be realized by integrated measurement method combined with the other perceptual devices.

The proposed technique will be improved not only to the engineering applications but the medical ones, such as the bio-feedback system in rehabilitation or the phyisical support system for handicapped persons.

## Author details

Takeshi Tsujimura
*Department of Mechanical Engineering, Saga University, Japan*

Sho Yamamoto
*Department of Mechanical Engineering, Saga University, Japan*

Kiyotaka Izumi
*Department of Mechanical Engineering, Saga University, Japan*

## 7. References

Chan, F. H., Lam, Y. Y., Zhang, Y., & Parker, P. A. (2000). Fuzzy EMG classification for prosthesis control, *IEEE Transactions on Rehabilitation Engineering*, Vol. 8, No. 3, (2000), pp. 305–311

Chen, X., Zhang, X., Zhao, Z., Yang, J., Lantz, V., & Wang, K. (2007). Multiple Hand Gesture Recognition based on Surface EMG Signal, *The 1st International Conference on Bioinformatics and Biomedical Engineering 2007,*(2007), pp.506-509

Fukuda, O., Tsuji, T., Kaneko, M., & Otsuka, A. (2003). A human-assisting manipulator teleoperated by EMG signals and arm motions, *IEEE Transactions on Robotics and Automation,* Vol. 19, No. 7, (2003), pp. 323–345

Graupe, D., Magnussen, J., & Beex, A. A. M. (1978). A micro-processor system for multifunctional control of upper limb prostheses via myoelectric signal identification, *IEEE Transactions on automatic control,* Vol. 23, No. 4, (1978), pp. 538–544

Huang, Y., Englehart, K.B., Hudgins, B., & Chan, A.D.C. (2005). A gaussian mixture model based classification scheme for myoelectric control of powered upper limb prostheses, *IEEE Transactions on Biomedical Engineering,* Vol. 52, No. 11, (2005), pp.1801-1810

Hudgins, B., Parker, P. A., & Scott, R. N. (1993). New strategy for multi-function myoelectric control, *IEEE Transactions on Biomedical Engineering,* Vol. 40, No. 1, (1993), pp. 82–94

Ibe, A., Gouko, M., & Ito K. (2009). Discrimination of Combined Motions for Prosthetic Hands Using Surface EMG Signals, *Transactions of the Society of Instrument and Control Engineers,* Vol. 45, No. 12, (2009), pp.717-723

Jacobson, S. C., Knutti, D. F., Johnson, R. T., & Sears, H. H. (1982). Development of the utah artificial arm, *IEEE Transactions on Biomedical Engineering,* Vol. 29, No. 4, (1982), pp. 249–169

Karlik, B., & Tokhi, M. O. (2003). A fuzzy clustering neural network architecture for multifunction upper-limb prosthesis, *IEEE Transactions on Biomedical Engineering,* Vol. 50, No. 11, (2003), pp. 1255–1261

Milner-Brown, H. S., & Stein, R. B. (1975). The relation between the surface electromyogram and muscular force, *Journal of Physiology,* Vol. 246, (1975), pp. 549–569

Oskoei, M.A., & Huosheng, H. (2008). Support Vector Machine-Based Classification Scheme for Myoelectric Control Applied to Upper Limb, *IEEE Transactions on Biomedical Engineering,* Vol. 55, Issue 8, (2008), pp.1956 - 1965

Tsujimura, T., Yamamoto, S., & Izumi K. (2011). Finger Gesture Estimation Based on Forearm Electromyogram Signals, *7th International Symposium on Image and Signal Processing and Analysis,* (2011), pp. 113-118

Yamamoto, S., Tsujimura, T., & Izumi K. (2012). Hand gesture identification using forearm surface EMG signals, *Proc. of 2012 JSME Conference on Robotics and Mechatronics,* (2012), A1A-V06

Yoshikawa, M., Mikawa, M., & Tanaka, K. (2007). A myoelectric interface for robotic hand control using support vector machine, *IEEE /RJS International Conference on Intelligent Robots and Systems,* San Diego, (2007), pp.2723-2728

Yoshikawa, M., Mikawa, M., & Tanaka, K. (2009). Real-Time Hand Motion Classification Using EMG Signals with Support Vector Machines, *The IEICE Transactions on information and systems (Japanese edition)*, Vol.J92-D, No.1, (2009), pp.93-103

# Chapter 7

# Design and Control of an EMG Driven IPMC Based Artificial Muscle Finger

R.K. Jain, S. Datta and S. Majumder

Additional information is available at the end of the chapter

## 1. Introduction

The medical, rehabilitation and bio-mimetic technology demands human actuated devices which can support in the daily life activities such as functional assistance or functional substitution of human organs. These devices can be used in the form of prosthetic, skeletal and artificial muscles devices (Andreasen et al., 2005; Bitzer & Smagt, 2006; DoNascimento et al., 2008). However, we still have some difficulties in the practical use of these devices. The major challenges to overcome are the acquisition of the user's intention from his or her bionic signals and to provide with an appropriate control signal for the device. Also, we need to consider the mechanical design issues such as lightweight and small size with flexible behavior etc (Arieta et al., 2006; Shenoy et al., 2008). For the bionic signals, the electromyography (EMG) signal can be used to control these devices, which reflect the muscles motion, and can be acquired from the body surface. We are familiar with the fact that ionic polymer metal composite (IPMC) has tremendous potential as an artificial muscle. This can be stimulated by supplying a small voltage of ±3V and shows evidence of a large bending behavior (Shahinpoor & Kim, 2001; 2002; 2004; Bar-Cohen, 2002). In place of the supply voltage from external source for actuating an IPMC, EMG signal can be used where EMG electrodes show a reliable approach to extract voltage signal from body (Jain et al. 2010a; 2010b; 2011). Using this voltage signal via EMG sensor, IPMC can illustrate the bio-mimetic behavior through the movement of human muscles. Therefore, an IPMC is used as an artificial muscle finger for the bio-mimetic/micro robot.

The main objective of this chapter is to discuss the design and control of an IPMC based artificial muscle finger where this finger is actuated by EMG signal via movement of human finger. The movement is sensed by EMG sensor which provides signal for actuating the IPMC. When designing IPMC artificial muscle finger based micro gripper for handling the light weight components in an assembly, IPMC bending behaviour is utilized to hold the object. During holding the object, stable EMG signal is required. For this purpose, stable EMG signal is sent through proportional–integral–derivative (PID) controller to the system. Experimentally, it is found that IPMC based artificial muscle finger achieves similar movement like human index finger. This IPMC based artificial muscle finger attains deflection upto 12 mm. By developing a prototype of IPMC artificial muscle finger based micro gripper, it is demonstrated that EMG driven system like IPMC artificial muscle finger based micro gripper can be applicable in handling of light weight components. The major advantages of such system are that IPMC based artificial muscle finger tip shows the compliant behavior and consumes less energy for actuation. Therefore, EMG driven system shows enough potential to substitute for conventional mechanism in micro manipulation and rehabilitation technology.

This chapter is organized as follows: Section 2 describes the prior research related to EMG applications in robotics and bio-mimetics. Section 3.1 explains the basic design of IPMC artificial muscle finger based micro gripper which is driven by EMG signal. The basic tendon of index finger is studied in section 3.2 where muscles are identified for actuation of IPMC based artificial muscle finger. In section 3.3, a model for controlling the EMG signal is highlighted. Different types of control system are implemented for achieving stable data from EMG signal via index finger which is sent to IPMC based artificial muscle finger. Section 4 discusses experimental testing setup for activation of IPMC based artificial muscle finger by human finger through EMG. In section 5, the results are discussed and the conclusions are drawn in section 6. The future work is recommended in section 7.

## 2. Prior research related to EMG applications

In the past, some researchers have reported work related to shape memory alloy (SMA) and other similar actuators to develop the bio-mimetic fingers but IPMC artificial muscle based finger related work is limited. Pfeiffer et al. (1999) have designed artificial limbs and robot prostheses that are lightweight, compact and dexterous. This mimics the human anatomy and maintains a high lifting capability. EMG control is used for SMA actuated fingers in robot prostheses. DeLaurentis & Mavroidis (2002) have discussed the design of a 12 degree-of-freedom (DOF) SMA actuated artificial hand where the SMA wires are embedded intrinsically within the hand structure. Cocaud & Jnifene (2003) have investigated the use of artificial muscles as SMA actuators for robot manipulators. A solution is established in order to determine the optimal position of a muscle in various musculoskeletal configurations. Herrera et al. (2004) have also designed and constructed a prosthesis where linear actuators are used for designing the mechanical system and EMG sensors are introduced for designing the electrical control system. Bundhoo et al. (2005, 2008) have reported the design of artificially actuated finger by SMA towards development of bio-mimetic prosthetic hands. Different finger joints are actuated through SMA wires via EMG and the relationship between elongation/contraction of the SMA wires & the finger joints have been obtained. O'Toole & McGrath (2007) have also focused on mechanical design of a 12 DOF SMA actuated artificial hand. The SMA material is used for combination of high strength polymers such as polytetrafluoroethylene (PTFE), polyether ether ketone (PEEK) and low density metals such as titanium. Lau (2009) have carried out research work on a design and development of an intelligent prosthetic hand based on hybrid actuation through DC motor & SMA wires. These are controlled by myoelectric signal. Two novel features are introduced in the new prosthetic hand. Firstly, its hybrid actuation mechanism has the advantage of increasing the active degrees of freedom and secondly, using only two myoelectric sensors, has the potential for controlling more than three patterns of fingers movements. Pittaccio & Viscuso (2011) have developed a SMA wire device for the rehabilitation of the ankle joint where active orthosis powered by two rotary actuators like, NiTi wire are used to obtain ankle dorsiflexion and EMG signal is used to control the orthosis and trigger activation from muscle. Stirling et al. (2011) have shown the potential of SMA wire for an active, soft orthotic in the knee where NiTi based SMA wires is also used. A prototype is tested on a suspended, robotic leg to simulate the swing phase of a typical gait. Thayer & Priya (2011) have designed a biomimetic dexterous humanoid hand where the dexterity of the DART hand have been measured by quantifying functionality and typing speed on a standard keyboard. The hand consists of 16 servo motors dedicated to finger motion and three motors for wrist motion where some of joints are activated through SMA wires.

Some of the researchers have focused on the design of a biomechatronic robotic hand using EMG. Cheron et al. (1996) have found the relationship between EMG and the arm kinematics through dynamic recurrent neural networks (DRNN) method whereas Hudgins et al. (1997) have focused on a new control scheme, based on the recognition of naturally myoelectric signal patterns, transfers the burden of multifunction myoelectric control from the amputee to the control system. Rosen et al. (2001) have developed a myosignal-based exoskeleton system. This is implemented in an elbow joint, naturally controlled by the human. The human–machine interface is set at the neuromuscular level, by using the neuromuscular signal (EMG) as the primary command signal for the exoskeleton system. The EMG signals along with the joint kinematics are fed into a myoprocessor (Hill-based muscle model) which in turn predicts the muscle moments on the elbow joint. Banks (2001) has given remarkable effort towards design and control of an anthropomorphic robotic finger with multi-point tactile sensation whereas Light et al. (2002) have emphasized on intelligent multifunction myoelectric control of hand prostheses. Peleg et al. (2002) have extracted multiple features via EMG signal from hand amputees which is selected by help of a genetic algorithm. Fukuda et al. (2003) have developed a prosthetic hand where human-assisting manipulator system based on the EMG signals is utilized. Wheeler (2003) has presented a neuro-electric interface method for virtual device control. The sampled EMG data is taken from forearm and then is fed into pattern recognition software that has been trained to distinguish gestures from a given gesture set. Krysztoforski et al. (2004) have given remarkable effort towards recognition of palm finger movements on the basis of EMG signals with the application of wavelets.

Crawford et al. (2005) have used EMG signals for classifying in real-time with an extremely high degree of accuracy in a robotic arm-and-gripper. A linear support vector machines (SVM) based classifier and a sparse feature representation of the EMG signal are used.

Hidalgo et al. (2005) have proposed a design of robotic arm employing fuzzy algorithms to interpret EMG signals from the flexor carpi radialis, extensor carpi radialis and biceps brachii muscles. The control and acquisition systems are composed of a microprocessor, analog filtering, digital filtering & frequency analysis, and finally a fuzzy control system. Mobasser & Hashtrudi-Zaad (2005) have estimated rowing stroke force with EMG signal using artificial neural network method from upper arm muscles which is involved in elbow joint movement, sensed elbow angular position and velocity. Gao et al. (2006) have focused on acquiring the data from the upper limb of the body for robotic arm motion using EMG whereas Frigo et al. (2007) have detected EMG signal from voluntarily activated muscles which is controlled for functional neuromuscular by electrical stimulation. A comb filter (with and without a blanking window) is applied to remove the signal components synchronously correlated to the stimulus. Roy et al. (2007) have compared the performance of different sEMG signal at various conditions. These performances depend on the electro-mechanical stability between the sensor and its contact with skin. Zollo et al. (2007) have put a remarkable effort on the control system of biomechatronic robotic hand and on the optimization of the hand design in order to obtain human like kinematics and dynamics. By evaluating the simulated hand performance, the mechanical design is iteratively refined. The mechanical structure and the ratio between numbers of actuators to the number of DOF have been optimized. Yagiz et al. (2007) have developed a dynamic model of the prosthetic finger where a non chattering robust sliding mode control is applied to make the model follow a certain trajectory. Wege & Zimmermann (2007) have shown the potential of EMG control for a hand exoskeleton device. The device has been developed with focus on support of the rehabilitation process after hand injuries or strokes. Itoh et al. (2007) have studied the hand finger operation using sEMG during crookedness state of the finger. Two electrodes (Ag/AgCl electrodes) are sticked randomly on the forearm muscles and the intensity of EMG signals at different muscles is measured for each crooked finger.

Hao et al. (2008) have studied the design of pneumatic muscle actuator based robotic hand where its compliance and dexterity handling are attempted. A single finger is controlled by fuzzy & PID controller and comparative studies are discussed. Murphy et al. (2008) have explored the micro electro-mechanical systems based sensor for mechanomyography system whereas Saponas et al. (2008) have also explored the feasibility on muscle-computer interaction methodology that directly senses and decodes human muscular activity rather than relying on physical device actuation or user actions. Andrews (2008) has determined an effective approach to finger movement classification in typing tasks using myoelectric data which are collected from the forearm. Cesqui et al. (2008) have explored the use of EMG signals for post-stroke and robot-mediated therapy. In this work, a pilot study has been reported under young and healthy subjects where experiments are conducted to determine whether it is possible to build a static map to cluster EMG activation patterns for horizontal reaching movements. Chen et al. (2008) have implemented an EMG feedback control method with functional electrical stimulation cycling system (FESCS) for stroke patients. The stroke patients often suffer from low limbs paralysis. By designing the feedback control protocol of FESCS, the physiological signal is recorded with help of FPGA biomedical module, DAC and electrical stimulation circuit. Lee et al. (2009) have described a development procedure of bio-mimetic robot hand and its control scheme where each robot hand has four under-actuated fingers, which are driven by two linear actuators coupled together. Dalley et al. (2009) have given emphasis of an anthropomorphic hand prosthesis that is intended for use with a multiple-channel myoelectric interface. The hand contains 16 joints, which are differentially driven by a set of five independent actuators. Hu et al. (2009) have presented a comparison between electromyography-driven robot and passive motion device on wrist rehabilitation for chronic stroke patients. By comparative study, it was found that the EMG-driven interactive training had a better long-term effect than the continuous passive movement (CPM) treatment.

Blouin et al. (2010) have focused on control of arm movement during body motion as revealed by EMG whereas Luo & Chang (2010) have explored a feasibility study on EMG signal integrated with multi-finger robot hand control for massage therapy applications. The forearm EMG of a person massaged by the human hands is recorded and analyzed statistically. Khokhar et al. (2010) have showed the potential of EMG applications where SVM classification technique is suitable for real-time classification of sEMG signals. This technique is effectively implemented for controlling an exoskeleton device. Huang et al. (2010) have designed a robust EMG sensing interface for pattern classification. The aim of this study was to design sensor fault detection (SFD) module through the sensor interface to provide reliable EMG pattern classification. This module monitors the recorded signals from individual EMG electrodes and performs a self-recovery strategy to recover the classification performance when one or more sensors are disturbed. Naik et al. (2010) has studied the pattern classification of myo-electric signal during different maximum voluntary contractions using BSS techniques for a blind person whereas Artemiadis & Kyriakopoulos (2010 & 2011) have presented a switching regime model for the EMG-based control of a robot arm where decode the EMG activity of 11 muscles has a continuous representation of arm motion in the 3-D space. The switching regime model is used to overcome the main difficulties of the EMG-based control systems, i.e. the nonlinearity of the relationship between the EMG recordings and the arm motion, as well as the non-stationary of EMG signals with respect to time. Vogel et al. (2011) have demonstrated the robotic arm/hand system that is controlled in real time in 6 dimension Cartesian space through measured human muscular activity via EMG. DLR Light-weight Robot III is used during demonstration of impedance control. Li et al. (2011) have presented a robot control system using four different gestures from an arm. These are achieved by EMG signal using phase synchrony features. The phase synchrony analysis using the recent multivariate extensions of empirical mode decomposition (MEMD) is carried out. Joshi et al. (2011) have focused on brain-muscle-computer interface using a single sEMG signal. Initial results show that the human neuromuscular system can simultaneously manipulate partial power in two separate frequency bands of a sEMG power spectrum at a single muscle site. Matsubara et al. (2011) have proposed an interface to intuitively control robotic devices using myoelectric signals. Through learning procedure, a set of myoelectric signals is captured from multiple subjects in the system and it can be used as an adaptation procedure to a new user after only a few interactions.

Recently, Ahmad et al. (2012) have presented a review report on different techniques of EMG data recording where condition of an ideal pre-amplifier, signal conditioning and its amplification are discussed. Sun et al. (2012) have conducted an isokinetic exercise to realize the characteristics of femoral muscles in human knee movement through EMG where a mechanical model of muscle for human knee movement is established. Qi et al. (2012) have developed algorithms for muscle-fatigue detection and muscle-recruitment patterns in routine wheel chair propulsion scenarios, e.g., daily practice where for analysis purpose two speeds of muscular behavior are chosen. Gandole (2012) has developed an artificial intelligent model using focused time lagged recurrent neural network (FTLRNN) method with a single hidden layer. FTLRNN method reduces noise intelligently from the EMG signal. Chan et al. (2012) have developed an assessment platform for upper limb myoelectric prosthetic devices using EMG. The assessment platform consists of an acquisition module, a signal capture module, a programmable signal generation module and an activation & measurement module. The platform is designed to create a sequence of activation signals from EMG data captured from a patient.

An EAP actuator based design for IPMC fingers have been discussed by Biddiss & Chau (2006). This shows the potential of electroactive polymeric sensors within an operating range of voltage (±3V) whereas Kottke et al. (2007) have reported on how to stimulate and activate a non-biological muscle such as an IPMC. Lee et al. (2006, 2007) have also demonstrated the potential of an IPMC actuating system with a bio-mimetic function using EMG signals. A mean absolute method is used for achieving the filtered EMG signal. Aravinthan et al. (2010) have designed a multiple axis prosthetic hand using IPMC. EMG signal through programmable interface controller (PIC) is sent to the IPMC prosthetic material to perform the required actions. By doing experiments, the potential of prosthetic hand using IPMC is shown. After that, we have also demonstrated actuation of IPMC through EMG via forearm muscles where  potential of IPMC based micro robotic arm has been shown for lifting the object (Jain et al., 2010a; 2010b; 2011; 2012). For further application of EMG driven system, we are discussing detailed analysis of EMG signal control point view of IPMC based artificial muscle finger for micro gripper in this chapter.

# 3. Design and control of IPMC based artificial finger driven by EMG signal

## 3.1. Basic design of IPMC artificial muscle finger based micro gripper using EMG

For designing an IPMC artificial muscle finger based micro gripper using EMG, an IPMC strip (Size 40 mm × 10 mm× 0.2 mm) that imitates human finger movement, is assumed to be artificial muscle finger. This is fixed with holder and another plastic based finger of similar size is made for supporting the micro object as shown in Fig. 1. When human index finger moves up and down, it creates potential difference by its movements. This potential difference is transferred through EMG electrodes into the artificial muscle finger so that this finger is able to move accordingly and hold the object. The main function of EMG electrode is to detect the voltage from human muscles since human muscles generate few milli-voltages when they are contracting or expanding during movement. For transferring this voltage signal to actuate the artificial muscle finger, it needs the amplification setup which is discussed in section 4. Therefore, IPMC based artificial muscle finger is activated using EMG and it allows holding an object for micro assembly operation.

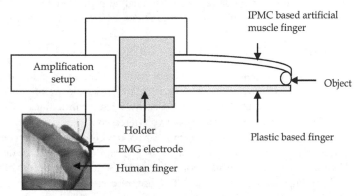

**Figure 1.** Schematic diagram of IPMC artificial muscle finger based micro gripper driven by EMG

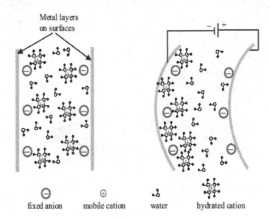

**Figure 2.** Schematic diagram of the actuation mechanism of IPMC (Chen et al., 2011)

During development of an EMG driven IPMC based artificial muscle finger, a typical IPMC strip (Procured custom made from Environmental Robots Inc., USA) is used which has a thin (approximately 200 μm) perfluorinated ion exchange base polymer membrane (Nafion-117) with metal electrodes of platinum (5–10 μm) fused on either side. As a part of the manufacturing process, this base polymer is further chemically coated with metal ions that comprise the metallic composites. It responds in wet/dry condition. An IPMC is usually kept in a hydrated state to ensure proper dynamic operation. When the material is hydrated, the cations will diffuse toward an electrode on the material surface under an applied electric field. Inside the polymer structure, anions are interconnected as clusters providing channels for the cations to flow towards the electrode (Chen et al., 2011). This motion of ions causes the structure to bend toward the anode as shown in Fig. 2. An applied electric field affects the cation distribution within the membrane, forcing the cations to migrate towards the cathode. This change in the cation distribution produces two thin layers, one near the anode and another near the cathode boundaries. The potential is generated by changing the potential electric field on cluster of ionic strips that provides the actuation of the strip.

## 3.2. Basic tendon of index finger for identification of EMG signal

To examine the bio-mimetic behavior of IPMC based artificial muscle finger, it is important to study the physiological structure of human finger. An internal structure of human index finger is shown in Fig. 3. The index finger is actuated by three intrinsic muscles and four extrinsic muscles. The intrinsic muscles consist of two interosseous (IO 1 and IO 2) muscles & one lumbrical (LU) muscle and four extrinsic muscles connected through long tendons i.e. extensor digitorum communis (EDC), extensor indicis proprius (EIP), flexor digitorum superficialis (FDS) and flexor digitorum profundus (FDP) (Bundhoo & Park, 2005). For heavy lifting & holding purpose, EDC and EIP are responsible in tendon network. Consequently, EMG electrodes are placed at these two positions on the human finger so that we can achieve direct actuation of IPMC based artificial muscle finger through said muscles.

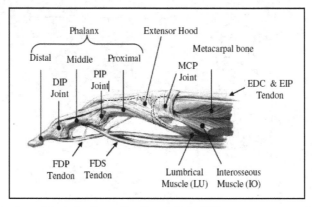

**Figure 3.** Basic tendons of the index finger (Bundhoo & Park, 2005)

## 3.3. Model for controlling the EMG signal for IPMC based artificial muscle finger

For acquiring the data from said muscles, EMG electrodes are placed for measuring the electric potential produced by voluntary contraction of muscle fiber on the human finger. The frequency range of the EMG signal is within 4 to 900 Hz. The dominant energy is concentrated in the range of 95 Hz and amplitude of voltage range is ±1.2 mV according to muscle contraction and the voltage function $V_{in}(t)$ in term of signal sample time ($t$) is given below,

$$V_{in}(t) = V_{ino}sin(2\pi ft) \tag{1}$$

Where, $V_{ino}$ is amplitude of EMG voltage (±0.0012 V); $f$ is frequency of EMG signal (95 Hz).

In Laplace domain, EMG input signal is written as

$$V_{in}(s) = \frac{2.96}{s^2 + 3.51e5} \tag{2}$$

Using these parameters, the circuit for filtered EMG signal is designed using MATLAB SIMULINK software as shown in Fig. 4.

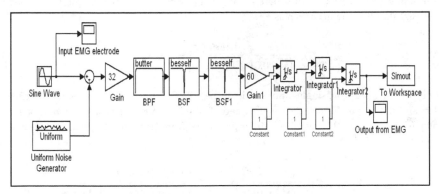

**Figure 4.** Block diagram of EMG signal behaviour from human index finger

In block diagram, the active EMG signal is taken from index finger muscle and uniform noise is considered. The electric potential is first amplified with gain 32 dB and then band pass filter (BPF) is used within specified frequency range (4 to 900 Hz). Using two band stop filters (BSF and BSF1), noise signal (60 Hz) that arises due to AC coupled power is eliminated. The signal is then passed through an amplifier with gain 60 dB. Subsequently, three integrators (Integrator, Integrator1 and Integrator2) are used for achieving better damped signal. The output of EMG signal with sampling time of $10^{-4}$ seconds after filtering is shown in Fig. 5.

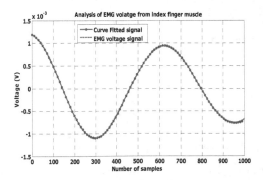

**Figure 5.** Acquired data from finger muscles via EMG signal

Thus, the total output duration of EMG signal for sampled data is 0.1 second. The general solution of acquired EMG voltage ($V_{EMG}$) through curve fitting method is obtained as given below,

$$V_{EMG}(t) = \sum V_0 sin(2\pi f_0 t + \delta_0), \quad 0 \le t \le 0.1 \tag{3}$$

where, $V_0$ is the amplitude of EMG voltage of sine function (±0.0012 V); $f_0$ is average frequency of sine function (4.7 Hz); $\delta_0$ is initial phase difference of sine function (1.66 rad); $t$ is signal sample time in second.

After adjustment of root mean square (RMS) value of this sine function, the EMG voltage $V_{EMGrms}(s)$ after filtering is written as

$$V_{EMG_{rms}}(s) = \frac{1.16e^{-5}(s^2 + 1.17e^{-4})}{\left(s^2 - 0.014s + 1.07e^{-4}\right)\left(s^2 + 0.014s + 1.07e^{-4}\right)} \tag{4}$$

For controlling purpose, single input single output (SISO) control system tool in MATLAB is used and the output $V_{EMG}(s)$ data is obtained. The initial overall transfer function of EMG voltage $V_{EMGinitial}(s)$ is obtained through output signal from (4) to input signal from (2) and is given as

$$V_{EMGinitial}(s) = \frac{3.92e^{-6}\left(s^2 + 1.17e^{-4}\right)\left(s^2 + 3.5e^5\right)}{\left(s^2 - 0.0146s + 1.07e^{-4}\right)\left(s^2 + 0.0146s + 1.07e^{-4}\right)} \tag{5}$$

After that, Nyquist criterion is applied to check the stability of EMG signal. The root-locus and bode scheme are plotted as shown in Fig. 6.

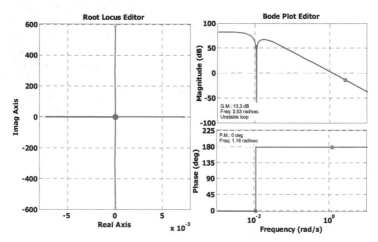

**Figure 6.** Root-locus and bode plot behaviour of EMG signal via finger in initial condition (Jain et al., 2011)

It is found that the zero-poles have real value on both sides of the real axis which does not meet the Nyquist stability criteria. Also from Fig. 6, gain cross-over frequency (GCF=2.53 rad/s) is greater than phase cross-over frequency (PCF=1.18 rad/s), indicating that this voltage obtained from EMG signal is unstable.

For achieving the stable EMG signal, different configurations of PID are analysed through SISO control tool of MATLAB software. By applying PD control with proportional control gain factor ($K_p$=1) and derivative control gain factor ($K_d$=1), EMG voltage $V_{EMGfinal\ 1}(s)$ is obtained as given below,

$$V_{EMGfinal1}(s) = \frac{(s^2+1.17e^{-4})(s^2+3.516e^5)}{(s+2.546e^5)(s^2-9.91e^{-9}s+1.17e^{-4})(s^2+1.38s+1.38)} \quad (6)$$

The root locus and bode plot are shown in Fig. 7. This indicates that the obtained data from EMG signal is unstable but through this control system the data is converging towards stability from initial condition.

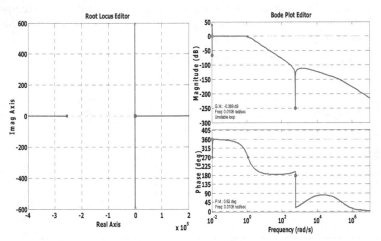

**Figure 7.** Root-locus and bode plot behaviour of human finger through PD controller

In case of PI controller, the unit proportional control gain factor ($K_p$=1) and integrator control gain factor ($K_i$=1) parameters are used. After applying this control system, EMG voltage $V_{EMGfinal\ 2}(s)$ is obtained as given below,

$$V_{EMGfinal2}(s) = \frac{3.92e^{-6}\ s\ (s^2+1.17e^{-4})\ (s^2+3.51e^5)}{(s+0.724)(s^2+9.91e^{-9}s+1.17e^{-4})(s^2-0.724s+1.90)} \quad (7)$$

The bode plot and root locus for this system are plotted as shown in Fig. 8. From this figure, it shows that the data from EMG signal is again unstable but the response has a better prospect of converging towards stability than previous configuration.

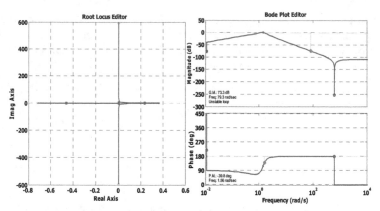

**Figure 8.** Root-locus and bode plot behaviour of EMG signal via finger through PI controller

After that, PID controller is used where proportional control gain factor ($K_p$= 0.5), integrator control gain factor ($K_i$= 1) and derivative control gain factor ($K_d$=1) are given in compensator to attain the stability of EMG voltage. For applying the PID control system, the SIMULINK block diagram is modified as shown in Fig. 9.

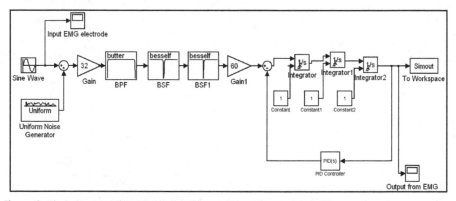

**Figure 9.** Block diagram of EMG signal via human finger after applying PID control system

Thereafter, the model is again simulated in MATLAB software, upon which, the data from finger muscles shows the all zero-poles in left hand side of real axis which satisfies the Nyquist criteria shown in Fig. 10. The final EMG voltage $V_{EMGfinal}$ (s) is acquired as given below,

$$V_{EMGfinal}(s) = \frac{s\left(s^2 + 1.17e^{-4}\right)\left(s^2 + 3.51e^5\right)}{\left(s + 2.54e^5\right)\left(s + 1.52\right)\left(s^2 + 1.83e^{-8}s + 1.17e^{-4}\right)\left(s^2 - 0.14s + 0.90\right)} \tag{8}$$

Also, GCF (1rad/s) is less than PCF (1.34 rad/s). Hence, a stable EMG voltage data is achieved. This filtered EMG signal is stable enough to provide necessary voltage signal across the IPMC for proper functioning during operation. The major advantage of this control system is that it is stable with least amount of noise. This signal is sent to artificial muscle finger for holding the object.

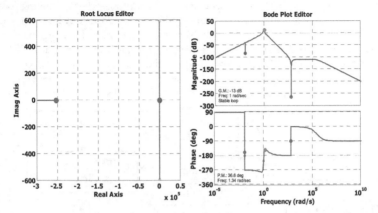

**Figure 10.** Root-locus and bode plot behaviour of EMG signal via finger through PID controller (Jain et al., 2011)

## 4. Experimental testing setup

In order to examine the bio-mimetic behaviour of IPMC based artificial muscle finger through EMG signal, EMG electrodes (Ag/Agcl based) are positioned at EDC and EIP muscles on the index finger. The input EMG signal from the muscle movement varies in the range of ±1.2mV (which is observed through oscilloscope). But activation of IPMC based artificial muscle finger needs the voltage of ±3V and current rating of 50-200 mA which is only possible by amplification of voltage and current. For desired output voltage to the artificial muscle finger, EMG signal is transferred through analog-digital convertor (ADC) card and PXI system (PXI-1031 along with NI-6289) in real time environment. EMG signal through electrodes are sent to an input channel at specified ports of the ADC card. Then this signal is amplified through amplification factor of 2550 using express VI of Labview 8.5 and sent to DAC output. But DAC output signal cannot provide enough current (50-200 mA) to drive an IPMC based artificial muscle finger. For achieving this current rating, the current amplification is done using customized IPMC control circuit by combining operational amplifier (Model: LM-324), transistor (Model: TIP 122) and resistances (1kΩ and 10Ω). Noise interference is eliminated by enabling low-pass filtering with PID control system to achieve the stability during operation of the artificial muscle finger as shown in Fig. 11. The IPMC size 40mm × 10 mm × 0.2 mm is used for testing purpose.

Now, in order to prevent the abrupt physio-chemical change of the IPMC nature and subsequent shortening of the actuation operating time of the IPMC material due to irreversible electrolysis (caused when the voltage applied across the two faces of an IPMC exceeds a maximum limit), two warning flags are used. One warning flag is placed at input EMG signal and another warning flag is placed at output voltage of DAC card where IPMC control circuit is connected. This limited voltage imposed on the IPMC based artificial muscle finger aborts the execution of the program when the warning flag has a high output. The flow chart for actuation of IPMC based artificial muscle finger is shown in Fig. 12. During operation, artificial muscle finger bends in a similar manner as that of the index finger. For generating force, this finger is held in cantilever configuration on the fabricated work bench. A load cell is used to collect the data at different angles of the index finger. The current and voltage analysis of the human muscles are also done through oscilloscope. Thus an IPMC artificial muscle finger based micro gripper driven by EMG is developed and the holding behaviour is demonstrated.

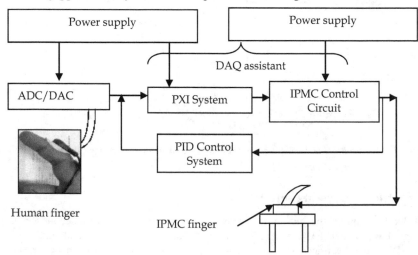

**Figure 11.** Basic testing layout for actuation of IPMC based artificial muscle finger

## 5. Results and discussion

During experimentation, the input parameter from muscle ranging from ±1.2 mV is taken through referenced single-ended (RSE) signal along with continuous sampled pulses. These pulses are amplified with the help of a PXI system (amplification factor 2550). The desired output voltage range is generated through a DAC output port. The output signal is connected to IPMC based artificial muscle finger. Due to amplified output voltage from the DAC, an IPMC strip bends in one direction for holding the object. By changing the movement of human finger in an opposite direction, reverse behaviour of IPMC is obtained. The characteristics of IPMC based artificial muscle finger are traced on a graph paper and plotted as shown in Fig. 13. It shows that IPMC based artificial muscle finger gives similar bending behaviour as a human finger (Fig. 14). It is also observed that the deflection of IPMC based artificial muscle finger changes with voltage upto 12 mm in one direction. When this finger moves reverse direction, the characteristic of artificial finger does not attempt the same behaviour. It shows the error between two paths is 0.5 mm. The deflection characteristic of IPMC based artificial muscle finger ($\delta$) in term of voltage ($V$) with cubic behaviour for holding is given below,

$$\delta(V) = 0.67 \times V^3 - 1.9 \times V^2 + 3.7 \times V - 0.17 \ \left(\text{in mm}\right) \tag{9}$$

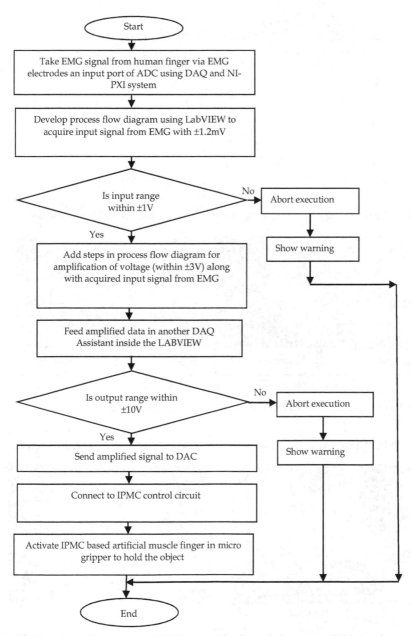

**Figure 12.** Flow chart of for actuation IPMC based artificial muscle finger using EMG signal

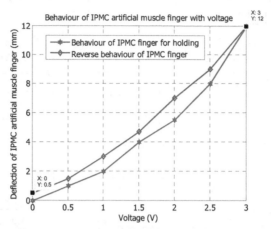

**Figure 13.** Deflection behaviour of IPMC based artificial muscle finger with different voltages

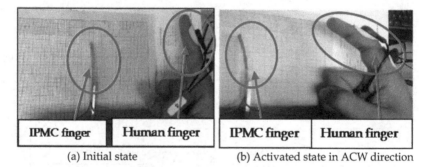

(a) Initial state                                    (b) Activated state in ACW direction

**Figure 14.** Control of IPMC based article muscle finger through EMG signal (Jain et al., 2011)

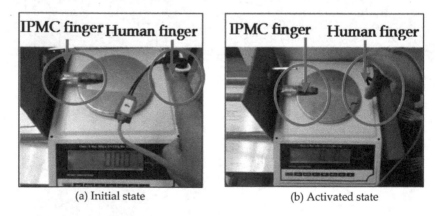

(a) Initial state                                    (b) Activated state

**Figure 15.** Load test setup for IPMC based artificial muscle finger using load cell

For generating force by the artificial muscle finger, a testing setup with load cell is used. The IPMC based artificial muscle finger is placed in cantilever mode, and a load cell is placed under the tip of the IPMC which produces the reactive force. When human finger moves downward, the generated force by IPMC artificial muscle finger increases accordingly in the load cell as shown in Fig. 15.

By controlling the movement of human finger, the generated force varies accordingly. The generated force characteristic with voltage shows a cubic polynomial behaviour as shown in Fig. 16 when IPMC artificial muscle finger touches the load cell. This happens due to compliant behaviour of IPMC. The generated force (F) by IPMC based artificial muscle finger in term of voltage (V) is given below,

$$F(V) = 0.11 \times V^3 + 0.25 \times V^2 + 1.6 \times V - 0.11 \quad \left( \text{in mN} \right) \tag{10}$$

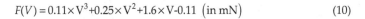

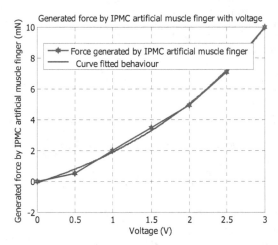

**Figure 16.** Generated force by IPMC based artificial muscle finger at tip with voltage

The maximum generated force of 10 mN is achieved by IPMC based artificial muscle finger at 45⁰ angle of index finger with cubic polynomial behaviour as shown in Fig. 17. This happens due to human finger behaviour where EIP and EDC muscles are connected with DIP and PIP joints. The generated force (F) by IPMC based artificial muscle finger at tip in term of human finger angle (θ) is also obtained as under

$$F(\theta) = -0.000083 \times \theta^3 + 0.01 \times \theta^2 - 0.063 \times \theta + 0.045 \quad \left( \text{in mN} \right) \tag{11}$$

For observing the real time IPMC based artificial muscle finger behaviour with moving human finger angle, experiments are conducted and data are plotted as shown in Fig. 18 and it shows almost proportional behaviour with quadratic relationship. This occurs due to human finger behaviour where EIP and EDC are connected with IO and LU muscles (Fig. 3).

The relationship between IPMC based artificial muscle finger displacement ($\delta$) and human finger angle ($\theta$) is given below,

$$\delta(\theta) = -0.0016 \times \theta^2 + 0.34 \times \theta - 0.15 \quad (\text{in mm}) \tag{12}$$

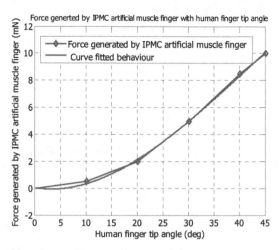

**Figure 17.** Generated force by IPMC based artificial muscle finger with human finger angle

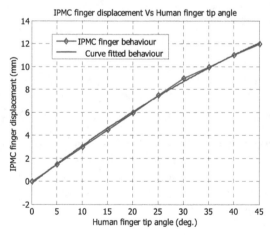

**Figure 18.** Relationship between IPMC based artificial muscle finger and human finger angle

For actuation of IPMC based artificial muscle finger, the analysis of activated muscles is carried out as given in Table 1. We have analysed different conditions during contraction of different muscles of index finger like intrinsic and extrinsic which are responsible for actuation of IPMC based artificial muscle finger so that they can be used to hold an object.

| Cases | Intrinsic muscles | | | Extrinsic muscles | | | | State | Polarity | |
|-------|------|------|------|------|------|------|------|-------|--------|--------|
|       | IO 1 | IO 2 | LU   | EDC  | EIP  | FDS  | FDP  |       | Side A | Side B |
| 1 | OFF | OFF | OFF | OFF | OFF | OFF | OFF | None | None | None |
| 2 | ON | OFF | ON | OFF | OFF | ON | ON | Adduction | +ive | -ive |
| 3 | OFF | ON | ON | ON | ON | OFF | OFF | Abduction | -ive | +ive |
| 4 | ON | ON | ON | ON | ON | ON | ON | None | None | None |

**Table 1.** Analysis of different condition of muscles

The two surfaces of IPMC are denoted as side A and side B. In case of intrinsic muscles, the adduction is possible. When IO 1 or IO 2 are in either "on" or "off" condition along with LU muscle in "on" condition then it shows the abduction state. In case of extrinsic muscles, EDC and EIP muscles both are in "off" condition to achieve the adduction state when FDS and FDP muscles both are in "on" condition and for attaining the abduction state EDC and EIP both are in "on" condition when FDS and FDP both are in "off" condition. In rest cases, no power is achieved. Therefore, IPMC based artificial muscle finger is activated in above mentioned conditions from muscles.

The voltage characteristic behavior is taken from EMG and fed to IPMC based artificial muscle finger for actuation in real time environment as shown in Fig. 19. It is found that the trend of IPMC actuation voltage is similar to EMG voltage with amplification factor.

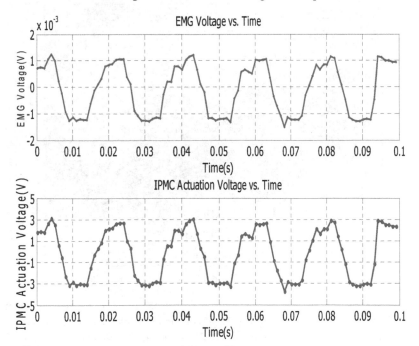

**Figure 19.** Different voltage responses in real time environment

The EMG voltage $V_{EMG}$ (t) and IPMC actuation voltage $V_{IPMC\ actuation}$ (t) equations are respectively given below,

$$V_{EMG}(t) = \sum V_{0E} sin(2\pi f_{0E} t + \delta_{0E}), \qquad 0 \le t \le 0.1 \qquad (13)$$

and

$$V_{IPMCactuation}(t) = \sum V_{0I} sin(2\pi f_{0I} t + \delta_{0I}), \qquad 0 \le t \le 0.1 \qquad (14)$$

Where, $V_{0E}$ is average value of EMG voltage (V); $f_{0E}$ is EMG frequency range (Hz) ; $t$ is signal sample time (s) ; $\delta_{0E}$ is phase difference when signal is taken through EMG (rad); $V_{0I}$ is average value of IPMC actuation voltage (V); $f_{0I}$ is IPMC actuation frequency range (Hz); $\delta_{0I}$ is phase difference when signal is given to IPMC (rad). For finding the frequency range of each signal, the experimental data are taken and solved through MATLAB curve fitting tool. The numerical values are $V_{0E}$= 0.001451±0.0002707 V, $f_{0E}$= 4.7±0.006201 Hz, $\delta_{0E}$= -1.736±0.036 rad, $V_{0I}$= 2.493±0.208, $f_{0I}$= 48.5±0.65 and $\delta_{0I}$= -10.5732±0.6556 rad. From these data, it is found that EMG frequency range ($f_{0I}$) is similar to simulated data and IPMC actuation frequency range is 48.5±0.65 Hz which is in between human muscle frequency range (48-52Hz).

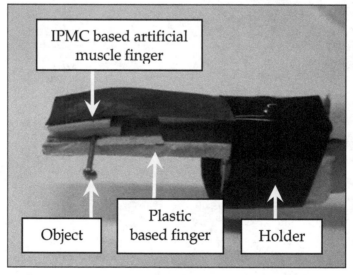

**Figure 20.** IPMC based artificial muscle finger based micro gripper driven by EMG

After these analyses, an IPMC artificial muscle finger based micro gripper is developed which is driven by EMG as shown in Fig. 20 where one IPMC based artificial muscle finger and other plastic based finger are fixed with double sided tape within one holder. The IPMC based artificial muscle finger is connected through copper tape and wire with EMG sensor so that an IPMC based artificial muscle finger is activated by EMG signal via human finger. The packing tape is also placed on the tip of IPMC based artificial muscle finger so that this finger perfectly holds the object like micro pin for assembly. After these observations, it is understood that IPMC finger behaves as an artificial muscle and this characteristic is implemented in the development of IPMC artificial muscle finger based micro gripper for holding the object through EMG. The major advantages of EMG-driven IPMC based artificial muscle finger are low voltage in man-machine interface, large bending amplitude and simple control that are applied in development of micro/bio robot.

## 6. Conclusion

In order to develop the micro/bio-mimetic robot for micro assembly, the potential of an EMG driven artificial finger is discussed in this chapter. An artificial finger for micro assembly is designed using IPMC where IPMC is used as an active artificial finger for holding the object. An IPMC has several advantages such as actuating through a small voltage (±3 V), light in weight, flexible in nature and does not involve sophisticated controllers for operation. For activating the IPMC based artificial finger, voltage is taken from human index finger through EMG sensor instead of battery source as this is used as a man-machine interface device. Principally, EMG sensor acquires the signal from body during expansion or contraction of muscles. These movements are transferred into an IPMC based artificial muscle finger. For achieving the stable data from EMG, different configurations of control methods are analysed. A PID control system is implemented for attaining the noiseless and stable signal from the user's myoelectric signal. While acquiring the data, a differential amplification technique is applied where data is filtered through a band pass filter and noise is eliminated through three band stop filters. For sending this signal to the IPMC, an algorithm has been developed in Labview software which gives emphasis on following points:

- Acquire voltage data (±1.2mV) from human index finger using EMG sensor through data acquisition system
- Amplify the continuous EMG signal through DAQ assistant enabling the filter and domain frequency range options
- Activate IPMC finger through amplified data (±3V) using interface device for functioning as artificial muscle finger

Experimentally, it is demonstrated that IPMC based artificial muscle finger is capable of adopting this voltage from EMG signal and mimics as a human finger. From application point of view, an IPMC artificial finger based micro gripper is developed and its capability is also verified. Through this demonstration, it is proved that IPMC can be activated through EMG signal and is applicable as flexible and compliant finger for holding the object in the fields of micro manipulation. IPMC based artificial muscle could also be a replacement of an electro-mechanical system like electric motors in the application field of rehabilitation technology.

## 7. Future direction

In future, we will focus on developing well equipped EMG driven micro robotic system where IPMC based micro robotic arm along with multiple IPMC artificial fingers will be used. IPMC based micro robotic arm will be operated through human fore arm movement for lifting and manipulation. Multiple IPMC fingers will be used for robust application like grasping, holding and mimicking of a human hand. Therefore, this new generation of robotic system can be really operated in real world through humans using EMG signals.

## Author details

R.K. Jain*, S. Datta and S. Majumder
*Design of Mechanical System Group/Micro Robotics Laboratory,*
*CSIR-Central Mechanical Engineering Research Institute (CMERI),*
*Durgapur, West Bengal, India*

## Acknowledgement

The authors are grateful to the Director, Central Mechanical Engineering Research Institute (CMERI), Durgapur, West Bengal, India for providing the permission to publish this book chapter. This work is financially supported by the Council of Scientific and Industrial Research (CSIR), New Delhi, India under eleventh five year plan on "Modular Re-configurable Micro Manufacturing System (NWP-30)".

## 8. References

Ahmad I., Ansari F. & Dey U. K. (2012). A review of EMG recording technique, *International Journal of Engineering Science and Technology,* Vol. 4, No. 2, pp. 530-539.

Andreasen D. S., Allen S. K. & Backus D. A. (2005). Exoskeleton with EMG based active assistance for rehabilitation, *Proceedings of the 2005 IEEE 9th International Conference on Rehabilitation Robotics,* Chicago, IL, USA, June 28 - July 1, pp. 333-336.

Andrews J. (2008). Finger movement classification using forearm EMG signals, *MS Thesis,* Queen's University, Kingston Ontario, Canada.

Aravinthan P., GopalaKrishnan N., Srinivas P. A. & Vigneswaran N. (2010). Design, development and implementation of neurologically controlled prosthetic limb capable of performing rotational movement, *IEEE International Conference RFID 2010,* Orlando, USA, 14-16April, pp. 241-244.

Arieta H., Katoh R., Yokoi H. & Wenwei Y. (2006). Development of a multi-DOF electromyography prosthetic system using the adaptive joint mechanism, *ABBI 2006,* Vol. 3, No. 2, pp. 1-10.

---

* Corresponding Author

Artemiadis P. K. & Kyriakopoulos K. J. (2010). EMG-based control of a robot arm using low-dimensional embeddings, *IEEE Transactions on Robotics*, Vol. 26, No. 2, pp. 393-398.

Artemiadis P. K. & Kyriakopoulos K. J. (2011). A switching regime model for the EMG-based control of a robot arm, *IEEE Transactions on Systems, Man and Cybernetics—Part B: Cybernetics*, Vol. 41, No. 1, pp. 53-63.

Banks J. L. (2001). Design and control of an anthropomorphic robotic finger with multi-point tactile sensation, *MS Thesis*, Artificial Intelligence Laboratory Massachusetts Institute of Technology.

Bar-Cohen Y. (2002). Electro-active polymers: current capabilities and challenges, *Proceedings of the SPIE Smart Structures and Materials Symposium EAPAD Conference* San Diego CA, 18-21 March, paper no 4695-02.

Biddiss E. & Chau T. (2006). Electroactive polymeric sensors in hand prostheses: bending response of an ionic polymer metal composite, *J. of Medical Engineering & Physics*, Vol. 28, pp. 568-578.

Bitzer S. & Smagt P. V. (2006). Learning EMG control of a robotic hand: towards active prostheses, *Proceedings of the 2006 IEEE International Conference on Robotics and Automation*, Orlando, Florida.

Blouin J., Guillaud E., Bresciani J. P., Guerraz M. & Simoneau M. (2010). Insights into the control of arm movement during body motion as revealed by EMG analyses, *J. of Brain Research*, Vol. 1309, pp. 40-52. Available: http:// www.sciencedirect.com

Bundhoo V. & Park E. J. (2005). Design of an artificial muscle actuated finger towards biomimetic prosthetic hands, *IEEE 12th International Conference on Advanced Robotics (ICAR)* Seattle WA, 18-20 July, pp. 368-370.

Bundhoo V., Haslam E., Birch B. & Park E. J. (2008). A shape memory alloy-based tendon-driven actuation system for biomimetic artificial fingers part I: design and evaluation, *J. of Robotica*, pp. 1-16.

Cesqui B., Krebs H. I. & Micera S. (2008). On the development of a new EMG–controlled robot-mediated protocol for post-stroke neurorehabilitation, *Proceeding ISG 08*. http://www.gerontechnology.info/Journal/Proceedings/ISG08/papers/130.pdf

Chan A., Kwok E. & Bhuanantanondh P. (2012). Performance assessment of upper limb myoelectric prostheses using a programmable assessment platform, *J. Med. Biol. Eng.*, (In press)

Chen C. C., Hsueh Y. H. & He Z. C. (2008). A Novel EMG Feedback Control Method in Functional Electrical Stimulation Cycling System for Stroke Patients, *World Academy of Science, Engineering and Technology*, Vol. 42, pp. 186-189.

Chen Z., Um T. I. & Smith H. B. (2011). A novel fabrication of ionic polymer–metal composite membrane actuator capable of 3-dimensional kinematic motions, *Sensors and Actuators*, Vol. A 168, pp. 131–139.

Cheron G., Draye J. P., Bourgeiosas M. & Libert G. (1996). A dynamic neural network identification of electromyography and arm trajectory relationship during complex movements, *IEEE Transactions on Biomedical Engineering*, Vol. 43, No. 5, pp. 552-558.

Cocaud C. & Jnifene A. (2003). Analysis of a two DOF anthropomorphic arm driven by artificial muscles, *Proceedings of the IEEE International Workshop on Haptic, Audio and Visual Environments and Their Applications (HAVE 2003)*, Ottawa, Ontario, Canada, September 21-22, pp. 37-42.

Crawford B., Miller K., Shenoy P. & Rao R. P. N. (2005). Real-time classification of electromyographic signals for robotic control, *Proceedings of AAAI*, pp. 523-528.

Dalley S. A., Wiste T. E., Withrow T. J. & Goldfarb M. (2009). Design of a multifunctional anthropomorphic prosthetic hand with extrinsic actuation, *IEEE/ASME Transactions on Mechatronics*, pp. 1-8.

DeLaurentis K. J. & Mavroidis C. (2002). Mechanical design of a shape memory alloy actuated prosthetic hand, *Technology and Health Care*, Vol. 10, pp. 91–106.

DoNascimento B. G., Vimieiro C. B. S., Nagem D. A. P. & Pinotti M. (2008). Hip orthosis powered by pneumatic artificial muscle voluntary activation in absence of myoelectrical signal, *Artificial Organs*, Vol. 32, No. 4, pp. 317–322, Blackwell Publishing, Inc. © 2008.

Frigo C., Ferrarin M., Frasson W., Pavan E. & Thorsen R. (2007). EMG signals detection and processing for on-line control of functional electrical stimulation, *J. of Electromyography and Kinesiology*, Vol. 10, pp. 351–360.

Fukuda O., Tsuji T., Kaneko M. & Otsuka A. (2003). A human-assisting manipulator teleoperated by EMG signals and arm motions, *IEEE Transactions on Robotics and Automation*, Vol. 19, No. 2, pp. 210-222.

Gandole Y. B. (2012). Noise reduction of biomedical signal using artificial neural network model, *International Journal of Engineering and Technology*, Vol. 2, No. 1.

Gao Z., Lei J., Song Q., Yu Y. & Ge Y. J. (2006). Research on the surface EMG signal for human body motion recognizing based on arm wrestling robot, *Proceedings of the 2006 IEEE International Conference on Information Acquisition*, Weihai Shandong China, 20-23 August, pp. 1269-1273.

Hao L., Wei F., Lin Y., Zheng P. & Tao W. (2008). Study on a new dexterous hand actuated by pneumatic muscle actuators, *Proceedings of the 7th JFPS International Symposium on Fluid Power* ,Toyama, 15-18 September, pp. 521-526.

Herrera A., Bernal A., Isaza D. & Adjouadi M. (2004). Design of an electrical prosthetic gripper using EMG and linear motion approach, *Florida Conference on Recent Advances in Robotics*, University of Central Florida.

Hidalgo M., Tene G. & Sánchez A. (2005). Fuzzy control of a robotic arm using EMG signals, *International Conference on Industrial Electronics and Control Applications*, pp. 1-6.

Hu X. L., Tong K. Y., Song R., Zheng X. J. & Leung W. F. W. (2009). A comparison between electromyography-driven robot and passive motion device on wrist rehabilitation for chronic stroke, *Neuro rehabilitation and Neural Repair*, Vol. 23, No. 8, pp. 837-846, http://nnr.sagepub.com.

Huang H., Zhang F., Sun Y. L. & H. Haibo (2010). Design of a robust EMG sensing interface for pattern classification, *J. Neural Eng.*, Vol. 7, 056005 (10pp).

Hudgins B., Englehart K., Parker P. & Scott R. N. (1997). A microprocessor-based multifunction myoelectric control system, *CMBE*, Institute of Biomedical Engineering University of New Brunswick Fredericton NB Canada. Available: http://www.ee.unb.ca/kengleha/papers/ CMBES97.

Itoh Y., Uematsu H., Nogata F., Nemoto T., Inamori A., Koide K. & Matsuura H. (2007). Finger curvature movement recognition interface technique using SEMG signals, *J. of Achievements in Materials and Manufacturing Engineering (JAMME)*, Vol. 23, No. 2, pp. 43-46.

Jain R. K., Datta S., Majumder S., A Paul & Banerjee P. (2012). Bio-mimetic behavior of IPMC using EMG signal for micro robot, *International Conference on Micro Actuators and Micro Mechanisms MAMM-2012*, CSIR-CMERI India, January 19-20.

Jain R. K., Datta S., Majumder S., Chowdhury S. & Banerjee P. (2011). IPMC artificial muscle finger activated through EMG. *Worldwide EAP newsletter on http://www.EAPnewsletter*. Vol. 13, No 01, June (The 25th issue), pp.10-12.

Jain R. K., Datta S., Majumder S., Mukherjee S., Sadhu D., Samanta S. & Benerjee K. (2010b). Bio-mimetic behaviour of IPMC artificial muscles using EMG signal, *ACEEE International Conference in Recent Technologies in Communication and Computing*, Kottyam India, 16-17 October, pp. 186-189.

Jain R. K., Dutta S. & Majumdar S. (2010a). Control of IPMC-based artificial muscle using EMG signal for hand prosthesis, *Worldwide EAP newsletter on http://www.EAPnewsletter*, Vol. 12, No 01, June (The 23th issue), pp.11-13.

Joshi S. S., Wexler A. S., Maldonado C. P. & Vernon S. (2011). Brain-muscle-computer interface using a single surface electromyographic signal: initial results, *Proceedings of the 5th International IEEE EMBS Conference on Neural Engineering*, Cancun, Mexico, 27April – 1 May, pp. 342-347.

Khokhar Z. O., Xiao Z. G. & Menon C. (2010). Surface EMG pattern recognition for real-time control of a wrist exoskeleton, *J. of Bio. Med. Eng.*, Vol. 9, No. 41, pp. 1-17.

Kim K. J. & Shahinpoor M. (2002). A novel method of manufacturing three dimensional ionic polymer metal composites (IPMCs) bio mimetic sensors actuators and artificial muscles, *Polymer*, Vol. 43, pp. 797-802.

Kottke E. A., Partridge L. D. & Shahinpoor M. (2007). Bio-potential activation of artificial muscles, *J. of Intelligent Material Systems and Structures*, Vol. 18, No. 2, pp. 103-109.

Krysztoforski K., Wolczowski A., Bedzinski R. & Helt K. (2004). Recognition of palm finger movements on the basis of EMG signals with the application of wavelets, *Task Quarterly*, Vol. 8, No. 2, pp. 269-280.

Lau B. G. (2009). An intelligent prosthetic hand using hybrid actuation and myoelectric control, *Ph D Thesis*, The School of Mechanical Engineering, University of Leeds.

Lee M. J., Jung S. H., Kim G. S., Moon I., Lee S. & Mun M. S. (2007). Actuation of the artificial muscle based on ionic polymer metal composite by electromyography (EMG) signals, *J. of Intelligent Material Systems and Structures*, Vol. 18, pp. 165-170. doi: 10.1177/1045389X06063463.

Lee M. J., Jung S. H., Lee S., Mun M. S. & Moon I. (2006). Control of IPMC-based artificial muscle for myoelectric hand prosthesis, *The First IEEE/RAS-EMBS International Conference on Biomedical Robotics and Biomechatronics BioRob 2006*, 20-22 February, pp. 1172-1177.

Lee S., Noh S., Lee Y. & Park J. H. (2009). Development of bio-mimetic robot hand using parallel mechanisms, *Proceedings of the 2009 IEEE International Conference on Robotics and Biomimetics*, Guilin China, 19 -23 December, pp. 550-555.

Li L., Looney D., Park C., Rehman N. U., & Mandic D. P. (2011). Power independent EMG based gesture recognition for robotics, *IEEE Engineering in Medicine and Biology Magazine*, pp. 793-796.

Light C. M., Chappell P. H., Hudgins B. & Englehart K. (2002). Intelligent multifunction myoelectric control of hand prostheses, *J. of Medical Engineering & Technology*, Vol. 26, No. 4, July/August, pp. 139-146.

Luo R. C. & Chang C. C. (2010). Electromyographic signal integrated robot hand control for massage therapy applications, *IEEE/RSJ International Conference on Intelligent Robots and Systems*, Taipei, Taiwan, October 18-22, pp. 3881-3886.

Matsubara T., Hyon S. H. & Morimoto J. (2011). Learning and adaptation of a stylistic myoelectric interface: EMG-based robotic control with individual user differences, *IEEE International Conference on Robotics and Biomimetics* (ROBIO), Phauket Island, Thailand, 7-11 December, pp. 390-395.

Mobasser F. & Hashtrudi-Zaad K. (2005). Rowing stroke force estimation with EMG signals using artificial neural networks, *IEEE International Conference on Control Application (CCA-2005)*, 28-31 August, pp. 825-830.

Murphy C., Campbell N., Caulfield B., Ward T. & Deegan C. (2008). Micro electro mechanical systems based sensor for mechanomyography, *19th International Conference on Bio-Signal*, Brno, Czech Republic.

Naik G. R., Kumar D. K. & Arjunan S. P. (2010). Pattern classification of myo-electrical signal during different maximum voluntary contractions: a study using BSS techniques, *Measurement Science Review*, Vol. 10, No. 1, pp. 1-6.

O'Toole K. T. & McGrath M. M. (2007). Mechanical design and theoretical analysis of a four fingered prosthetic hand incorporating embedded SMA bundle actuators, *World Academy of Science Engineering and Technology*, Vol. 31, pp. 142-149.

Peleg D., Braiman E., Yom-Tov E. & Inbar G. F. (2002). Classification of finger activation for use in a robotic prosthesis arm, *IEEE Transactions on Neural Systems and Rehabilitation Engineering*, Vol. 10, No. 4, pp. 290-293.

Pfeiffer C., DeLaurentis K. & Mavroidis C. (1999). Shape memory alloy actuated robot prostheses: initial Experiments, *Proceedings of IEEE International Conference on Robotics and Automation*, Vol. 3, pp. 2385-2391.

Pittaccio S. & Viscuso S. (2011). An EMG-controlled SMA device for the rehabilitation of the ankle joint in post-acute stroke, *Journal of Materials Engineering and Performance*, Vol. 20, No.4–5, pp. 666-670.

Qi L., Wakeling J., Grange S. & Ferguson-Pell M. (2012). Changes in surface electromyography signals and kinetics associated with progression of fatigue at two speeds during wheelchair propulsion, *JRRD*, Vol. 49, No. 1, pp. 23–34.

Rosen J., Brand M., Fuchs M. B. & Arcan M. (2001). A myosignal-based powered exoskeleton system, *IEEE Transaction on Systems, Man and Cybernetics—Part A: Systems and Humans*, Vol. 31, No. 3, pp. 210-222.

Roy S. H., Luca G. D., Cheng M. S., Johansson A., Gilmore L. D. & Luca C. J. D. (2007). Electro-mechanical stability of surface EMG sensors, *J. of Med. Bio. Eng. Comput.*, Vol. 45, pp. 447-457

Saponas T. S., Tan D. S., Morris D. & Balakrishnan R. (2008). Demonstrating the feasibility of using forearm electromyography for muscle-computer Interfaces, *CHI 2008*, Florence Italy, 5-10 April.

Shahinpoor M. & Kim K. J. (2001). Ionic polymer–metal composites: I. Fundamental, *Smart Materials Structure*, Vol. 10, pp. 819–833.

Shahinpoor M. & Kim K. J. (2004). Ionic polymer–metal composites: III. Modeling and simulation as biomimetic sensors actuator transducer and artificial muscles, *Smart Materials Structure*, Vol. 13, pp. 1362-1388.

Shenoy P., Miller K. J., Crawford B. & Rao R. P. N. (2008). Online electromyographic control of a robotic prosthesis, *IEEE Transactions on Biomedical Engineering*, Vol. 55, No. 3, pp. 1128-1135.

Stirling L., Yu C. H., Miller J., Hawkes E., Wood R., Goldfield E. & Nagpal R. (2011). Applicability of shape memory alloy wire for an active soft orthotic, *Journal of Materials Engineering and Performance*, Vol. 20, Issue 4-5, pp. 658-662.

Sun Y. P., Yen K. T., Kung H. K., Tsai Y. C., Lu K. C., Du C. M. & Liang Y. C. (2012). The muscular function for human knee movement revealed from electromyography: a preliminary study, *Life Science Journal*, Vol. 9, No. 1, pp. 453-456.

Thayer N. & Priya S. (2011). Design and implementation of a dexterous anthropomorphic robotic typing (DART) hand, *Smart Mater. Struct.*, Vol. 20, pp. 035010 (12pp).

Vogel J., Castellini C., & Smagt P. V. (2011). EMG-based teleoperation and manipulation with the DLR LWR-III, *IEEE/RSJ International Conference on Intelligent Robots and Systems*, San Francisco, CA, USA, September 25-30, pp. 672-678.

Wege A. & Zimmermann A. (2007). Electromyography (EMG) sensor based control for a hand exoskeleton, *Proceedings of the 2007 IEEE International Conference on Robotics and Bio-mimetics*, Sanya China, 15 -18 December, pp. 1470-1475.

Wheeler K. R. (2003). Device control using gestures sensed from EMG, *IEEE International Workshop on Soft Computing in Industrial Applications*, Binghamton University, Binghamton, New York, June 23-25, 2003.

Yagiz N., Arslan Y. Z. & Hacioglu Y. (2007). Sliding mode control of a finger for a prosthetic hand, *J. of Vibration and Control*, Vol. 13, No. 6, pp. 733–749, doi: 10.1177/1077546307072352.

Zollo L., Roccella S., Guglielmelli E., Carrozza M. C. & Dario P. (2007). Biomechatronic design and control of an anthropomorphic artificial hand for prosthetic and robotic applications, *IEEE/ASME Transactions on Mechatronics*, Vol. 12, No. 4, pp. 418-429.

# Chapter 8

# Application of Surface Electromyography in the Dynamics of Human Movement

César Ferreira Amorim and Runer Augusto Marson

Additional information is available at the end of the chapter

## 1. Introduction

Surface electromyography (sEMG) is a generic term for a method of recording electrical muscle activity. Numerous applications for this method have been developed in clinical practice, such as diagnosing neuromuscular diseases, analyzing and determining abnormalities or disorders and muscular rehabilitation (biofeedback) [3, 12, 27, 28].

sEMG is mainly used in the fields of physiotherapy, dentistry, physical education and biomechanics [12].

The duration of sEMG activity corresponds to the duration of muscle activation. The amplitude is the level of signal activity and varies with the amount of electrical activity detected in the muscle; it provides information about intensity of muscle activation. The observed sEMG frequency is due to a wide range of factors: muscle composition, characteristics of the action potential of the active muscles fibers, the intramuscular coordination process and electrode properties [22, 23, 28].

sEMG signals are also affected by the anatomical and physiological properties of the muscles, neuromuscular control of the peripheral nervous system and the instrumentation used to collect the signal.

The electronic EMG device amplifies, isolates and filters the electrical signal of muscles that occurs during muscle contraction. This signal must undergo conditioning to be captured [12].

A differential amplifier is, ideally, insensitive to noise and amplifies only the EMG signal, although in practice this is not the case. This situation occurs, first of all, because the noise that reaches the electrodes (inputs) doesn't necessarily have the same magnitude. Moreover, due to technological limitations, differential amplifiers cannot perfectly separate two-signal input.

The measurement that indicates the success of this separation is the common mode rejection ratio (CMRR), which is usually expressed in decibels (dB). The CMRR value of the differential amplifiers used in sEMG is on the order of 80 to 100 dB [3, 22, 24].

The sEMG equipment should be calibrated before recording signals. Calibration is important for fidelity, accuracy and reliability when reading the signal. The amplification factor is critical during the calibration process, since it is the ratio between the input voltage and that which comes out of the amplifier. The gain is selected according to the requirements of the type of experiment, the studied muscles, the type of electrodes involved and the planned use of the amplified signal. Whereas an sEMG signal has a maximum voluntary contraction amplitude not exceeding 5 millivolts (mV) peak-to-peak, the gain should be adjusted to 500-1000x [2,3,5].

During the mathematical processing of the sEMG signal, filters can be used to remove components that don't belong to the signal or components that are irrelevant for a given analysis.

The useful information in the sEMG signal is located in a particular frequency band (20-500 Hz), and is reduced by a filtering effect from the tissue located between the muscle fibers and the active sensing surface. The filter band corresponds to the frequency between the low- and high-cut filter frequencies [28].

Time-based signal processing can be carried out using a set of processing procedures intended to characterize the signal's curve and measure signal strength during the contraction. Signal processing applications in the time domain are widely used in areas such as neuromuscular coordination, motor control, the relationship between EMG and strength and muscular coordination in the dynamics of human movement.

This chapter will report, therefore, on the importance of sEMG with respect the dynamics of human movement [27].

## 2. Electromyography

The hypothesis that muscles generate electricity was by Francesco Redi in 1666 due to the suspicion that the discharges of electric fish were of muscular origin.

Along with other scientific developments during the Renaissance, interest in the muscles also began to increase. Leonardo da Vinci (1452 - 1519), for example, devoted careful attention to muscles and their anatomical function by conducting dissections of cadavers [12]

The main objectives of the first scientific experiments on muscles were to understand their structure and function [12]. A number of scientists since studied muscle dynamics. Luigi Galvani presented the first study on the electrical properties of muscles and nerves in 1791. He termed this neuromuscular potential "Animal Electricity". This discovery was recognized as the starting point for neurophysiology. Thereafter, a growing number of studies have been developed in this field [11]. sEMG is a technique for recording and monitoring the electrical signals from muscle contractions. A major methodological problem for EMG is the frequent presence of artifacts or noise. Artifacts or noise are defined as information whose origin is distinct from the neuroelectrical muscle activity signal. Some examples of this include interference, heart rate, poor contact between the electrode and the skin, etc.[12].

The presence of artifacts is difficult to avoid with this type of signal acquisition, since in order to amplify the signal, which is received in microvolts ($\mu$V), unwanted signals are also amplified and can compromise interpretation of the EMG signal. Thus, the signal-to-noise ratio has been a problem, and numerous studies have been undertaken to resolve EMG signal interpretation problems. After several attempts, a solution was found in the development of the differential amplifier [3] (ACIERNO, BARATTA & SOLOMONOW, 1995).

The signal amplifier is an electronic device that filters, amplifies and records bands of signals.

The initial problem with the amplifiers was that signal acquisition was dependent on the electrical resistance of the skin. Thus, in many studies skin resistance and temperature were initially monitored when the test was performed, conditions that made it difficult or impossible to reproduce and some EMG experiments [1].

Over time, corrections have been made to this system so that the amplifiers currently have high input impedance and attenuate noise levels, which allows the reproduction of experiments without interference with the results.

A main feature of this new generation of amplifiers is that they can amplify a particular type of biological signal independent of skin resistance [28]. The evolution of cables and connectors must also be considered in the development process of EMG acquisition equipment, since the type of conductive material and insulation system help minimize noise.

The main purpose of these developments is to help investigate and analyze human movement. The field of biomechanics is a practical example of the use of technological resources to interpret human movement [28].

Biomechanics can be defined generally as the study of the mechanics of living beings, or more specifically, the science that examines forces acting upon and within a structure and the biological effects produced by these forces [17]. Given the complex approach involved in biomechanics and human movement analysis [17], it is important to discuss the concepts, criteria and methods involved, focusing on the use of EMG for reliable interpretations.

EMG can be defined as the study of muscle function by analyzing the electrical signal generated during muscle contraction. Studying muscle function by means of EMG can be carried out under both normal and pathological conditions [12]. EMG has been used in important studies on muscle activity that have both qualitatively and quantitatively addressed the function of human movement. New information about muscle activity has been discovered as developments in processing and instrumentation have been applied to EMG [3,12, 15, 28] .

However, the purpose of this study is to present and discuss the use of sEMG as a quantification tool for studying motor and functional rehabilitation and neurophysiological abnormalities in the nervous system in comparison with peripheral stimuli.

Many authors have used different procedures to analyze EMG signals, which impedes both the comparison and reproducibility of results obtained in laboratory experiments, although their experiments have been described in internationally recognized scientific journals.

Thus, although there is diversity in the procedures for both applying EMG and analyzing the signals, this technique for investigating myoelectrical activity can be used in many different areas of study for different research purposes.

It is important, therefore, to demonstrate some of the applications of EMG as a research tool as well as different methods of analyzing EMG signals to facilitate the design of future and to foster appropriate analysis methods for signal data.

## 3. Kinesiological electromyography

The numerous applications of EMG include the diagnosis of neuromuscular disease or trauma in clinical practice, rehabilitation and the study of kinesiological muscle function in specific activities [2].

In one study [13] the EMG behavior of some of the major muscles of mastication was compared while subjects chewed different materials (two brands of chewing gum, cotton and parafilm) in order to identify the best material based on performance during bilateral chewing.

The EMG signal serves as an indicator of the initiation of muscle activity and can provide the firing sequence of one or more muscles involved in a specific task [12]. Information from the EMG signal is used to indicate the strength contributed by individual muscles and muscle groups.

In EMG, potentials are produced as a direct result of voluntary effort [18].

The electrodes used in EMG convert the electrical signal resulting from muscle depolarization into an electrical potential that can be amplified, and the difference in electrical potential can be processed. The potential amplitude depends on the difference in potential between the electrodes, such that the greater the potential difference, the greater the amplitude of the electrical potential or voltage [24].

The instrumentation used during the collection of EMG signals includes electrodes, amplifiers, filters, registers, decoders and sound equipment [27]. The choice of the electrode will depend on the muscle being studied.

The factors that influence the EMG signal can be divided into three categories: causes, determinants and intermediate factors [14].

Causative factors have an effect on the basic or elementary signal and are divided into extrinsic and intrinsic factors. Among the extrinsic factors are electrode configuration, the distance between the electrodes, the location of the electrodes over the motor point and the myotendonous junction, the location of the electrodes in relationship to the lateral border of the muscle and the orientation of the electrode in relation to muscle fibers. Intrinsic factors are the physiological, anatomical and biochemical characteristics of the muscle, such as the number of active motor units at the time a particular contraction occurs, the muscle fiber type, blood flow in the muscle, the fiber diameter, depth and location of the active fibers of the muscles in relation to the detection electrodes, the amount of tissue between the electrode and the muscle surface, as well as other factors such as the length of the depolarization zone and the ion flux across the membrane.

The intermediate factors are the physical and physiological phenomena that are influenced by one or more causative factors and, in turn, influence the determinants. Among this type are the detection electrode volume, the overlap of the action potential in the EMG signal, "cross-talk" with neighboring muscles, the conduction velocity of the action potential and the effect of spatial filtering. Since the determinant factors have a direct effect on the EMG signal and include the number of active motor units, the mechanical interaction between muscle fibers, the firing rate and the number of motor units detected, the amplitude, duration and shape of action potentials of motor units, as well as the recruitment and the stability of these units.

Soderberg and Cook described the limitations, collection methods and interpretation of electrical activity. Regarding the type of electrode, they believe that the sEMG can be used to analyze superficial muscles without causing discomfort to the volunteer [25].

The normalization procedure is usually considered necessary for recording, quantifying and comparing the EMG data obtained from different individuals or the same individual on different days [27].

Concern about the establishment of common standards for the collection, recording, analysis and interpretation of EMG signals has been expressed by a number of authors [12,27,28,], and more recently a practical guide for standardizing procedures to be used in EMG studies has been presented [1]. Thus, there is a tendency toward consensus among researchers on the use of appropriate instrumentation for collecting, recording and processing EMG signals.

Several studies [3, 5, 16, 27] have described the need to normalize the EMG signal amplitude when trying to make comparisons between different muscles, subjects, materials and days. This is due to the great variability observed in EMG tracings obtained from both different individuals and different muscles.

The EMG signal can be rectified by mathematical processing or by the root mean square (RMS) of squared instantaneous values . This signal can be passed through a low-pass filter for a presentation wrap the curve. Signal processing can then be carried out in accordance with the specific aim of the work [2]. In general, it is necessary to normalize the EMG signal in order to minimize the differences between individuals [16], when not comparing pre-and post-treatment.

## 4. Type and placement of electrodes

The electrodes available for kinesiological EMG are the passive and active surface type and the intramuscular type, each with its distinct characteristics, recommendations for use, advantages and disadvantages. The choice of electrode for capturing the EMG signal depends on the characteristics of the evaluated muscles. Thus, when analyzing certain muscles, size and location should be considered in the selection and application of electrodes [27].

The placement of surface electrodes is also another factor that influences the reliability of EMG recordings. The size, orientation and topography of electrodes influence EMG recordings [25].

Since the amplitude of the electrical potential is derived from the difference in potential observed between the electrodes, the inter-electrode distance should be controlled. Due to changes in distance, the same levels of contraction can result in different EMG signal amplitudes [24]. A major concern in sEMG is signal interference (cross-talk) from muscles surrounding the electrode. In one study [12], the surface electrodes were positioned on the midline of the muscle venter between the motor and the myotendonous junction with the detection surface towards the oriented fibers. However, this study was limited in that the electrodes were positioned between the motor and the myotendonous junction without electrically stimulating the motor points.

The surface area and shape of the electrode's contact surface as well as its location affect the signal amplitude, and the distance between the contact surfaces of the electrode affects the signal frequency. Figure 1 shows the characteristics of the EMG signal relative to the electrode position over the fibers. The most suitable location for electrode placement is in the direction of muscle fibers (Figure 2) and near the point of greatest electrical activity.

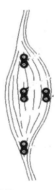

**Figure 1.** Representative signal results from different points in the muscle [3].

The electrodes must be carefully placed with regard to the adjacent muscles, since if the electrodes are too close to the other muscles then cross-talk may occur. Another important factor is the placement of the ground or reference electrode, which must have a good contact area.

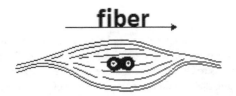

**Figure 2.** Diagram representing the placement of surface electrodes the direction of muscle fibers [3].

## 4.1. Considerations on the acquisition of EMG signals

EMG is a generic term for a method of recording the electrical activity of a muscle contraction. The numerous applications of electromyography (EMG) include diagnosing neuromuscular disease and determining the presence of dysfunctions or abnormalities in clinical practice, the rehabilitation of muscle action via EMG biofeedback, demonstrating kinesiology in anatomical studies, use in ergonomics as a tool for studying kinesiological muscle function related to posture and other biomechanical stress indicators, as well as a movement pattern identifier and a nervous system control parameter of the nervous system [28].

When interpreting the EMG signal for quantitative analysis, three fundamental characteristics can be distinguished: duration, amplitude and frequency, each of which is briefly described below [12].

The duration of EMG activity corresponds to the activation time of the selected muscle. The amplitude expresses the level of signal activity and varies with the amount of electrical activity detected in the muscle. It provides information on the intensity of muscle activation. RMS, average value, peak value and peak-to-peak value are ways of evaluating the amplitude of the signal. The frequency can be understood as the rate of excitation of the muscle cell. The frequency distribution of the EMG signal is due to a wide range of factors: muscle composition, the characteristics of the action potential of the active muscle fibers, the intramuscular coordination processes, the properties of the electrodes and their placement.

It can be said that signal processing begins, indirectly, as soon as the electrodes are placed. Electrode placement involves several factors that are decisive for the level and purity of the EMG signal to be collected, including: cleaning the skin, the amount and temperature of the conductive gel, the position of the electrodes and the signal-to-noise ratio, which expresses the balance between the energy of the signal generated during muscle contraction and the energy of noise from various undesirable sources [27].

The EMG signals are affected by anatomical and physiological muscle properties, peripheral nervous system control and the instrumentation used to collect the signal. Thus it is important to understand the basic muscle functions to correctly record EMG signals [12].

## 5. Biological amplifiers

In signal acquisition, analyzable information is obtained by studying the physical quantities involved in the activation process. These physical quantities can be measured by sensors that convert them into electrical signals and then record them using a data acquisition system (Figure 3). Computers make data acquisition more efficient and reliable and have the advantage of combining data storage with analysis and processing capability [21].

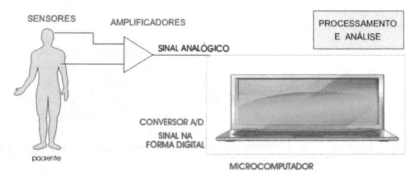

**Figure 3.** Diagram of a biological signal acquisition system [3].

Sensors and transducers are devices that convert physical quantities into electrical signals or current. Signal conditioners are electronic devices that modify the input signal in some way, whether by amplification, attenuation, filtering or isolation. The EMG signal, for example, enters at an amplitude of μV and must be amplified and filtered [3].

There are basically two techniques capturing an EMG signal: either monopolar or bipolar electrodes. In the monopolar configuration, only one electrode is placed on the skin over the muscle in question (Figure 4). This electrode detects the electrical potential relative to a reference electrode, which is placed in a location unaffected by the electrical activity generated by the analyzed muscle. In the bipolar configuration, two electrodes are used on the muscle as well as a reference (or ground) electrode placed in a neutral location (Figure 5). The human body is actually a good antenna for electromagnetic energy [3].

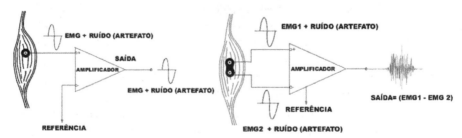

**Figure 4.** A) Schematic representation of a unipolar amplifier. B) Schematic representation of a bipolar amplifier [3].

## 6. Signal amplification

Gain is defined as the ratio between the voltage that enters and exits the amplifier. Gain should be selected to suit the characteristics of the experiment, the studied muscle, the electrode type and the use planned for the amplified signal. Considering that a sEMG signal has a maximum voluntary contraction amplitude not exceeding 5 mV peak-to-peak (Figure 6), the gain can be adjusted between 10 and 1000x. It is important to choose a gain that does not exceed at any stage the voltage expected from the system, or there will be a risk of either losing part of information or damaging the system itself [1].

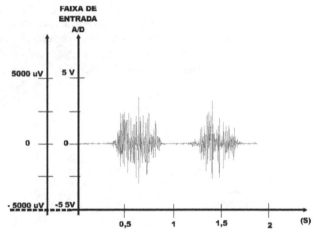

**Figure 5.** Appropriate gain range [3].

## 7. Signal filtering

Filters can be used to remove frequency components that do not belong to the signal or components that are irrelevant for a given analysis.

The captured signal can be filtered by hardware or software. Signal-filtering hardware can be used in the amplification step, while signal filtering by means of software can be performed during processing.

When using surface electrodes to measure EMG signals, interference from various sources can be mixed with the EMG signal. Each type of interference has its own characteristics that must be understood in order to remove it during the measurement phase or during processing. The useful information in the sEMG signal, which is a sum of the waves of varying frequency, is located between 20 and 500 Hz [12]. The signal is reduced due to the filtering effect of tissue located between the muscle fibers and the active sensing surface. The band pass filter corresponds to the frequency between the low frequency (high pass) and high frequency (low pass) cut-offs. Specific frequencies can also be filtered out with what are called "notch filters" [5, 11, 3, 23].

## 8. Analog-digital converter

An analog-digital (A/D) converter converts analog signals (EMG goniometry, force transducer) into digital data. The digitized signal can then be processed by the computer.

### 8.1. Input range and resolution of the A/D converter

The input range is a parameter associated with resolution and indicates the range of voltage that the A/D converter board can represent numerically. This band can be ± 5 V, ± 2.5 V, 0 to 5V, ± 10V etc.

When the input signals do not fall within the A/D card's range, it is necessary to condition them (amplify or attenuate) before inputting them into the A/D converter. Figure 6 shows an example in which the A/D converter or the conditioning gain is misaligned with the signal. Figure 7 depicts a gain adequate for visualizing the EMG signal.

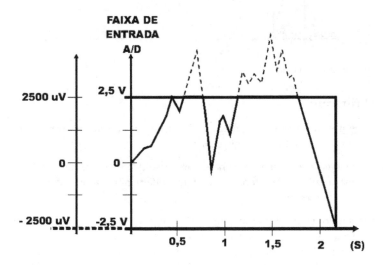

**Figure 6.** A/D converter range at odds with the amplification gain [3].

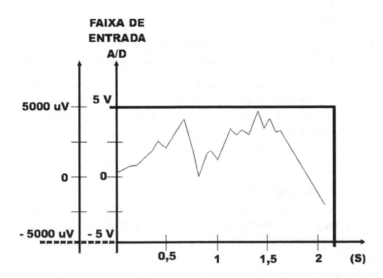

**Figure 7.** Properly aligned A/D converter range and amplification gain [3].

The resolution of an A/D converter indicates the lowest variation in analog signal that the converter can detect, which is generally presented in bits. Thus, converter resolutions can be 10, 12, 14 or 16 bits, etc., with the most common being 12- and 16-bit.

A converter with a 5V input range and a resolution of ± 12 bits can represent the input signal in 4096 (212) divisions and levels or detect changes of 2.4 mV (10 V divided by 4096 levels). A 16-bit converter may represent the same signal in 65536 (216) divisions and detect changes at levels of 153 μV. (10 V divided by 65,536 levels), [4].

## 8.2. Sampling rate

In practice, the input signal to the A/D converter varies over time; the goal is to record this variation. Since a computer's storage capacity is finite, the recording can only continue for a limited time.

The discretization of time is carried out by sampling the signal at regular intervals. The reverse of this interval is the sampling rate. For example, at a sampling rate of 100 samples per second (i.e., 100 Hz), the interval between samples is 10 ms. The sampling rate is equivalent to the resolution of the A/D conversion but applied to time.

However, due to the limited space available for data storage, there is a compromise between the sampling rate and the duration of acquisition. For example, for sampling rate of 100 samples per second, the maximum acquisition will be 166 minutes and 40 seconds. By increasing the rate to 1000 samples per second, the maximum is 16 minutes and 40 seconds.

The sampling rate must also be very low compared to the frequency of signal variation due to the effects of sub-sampling (aliasing).

An aliasing effect occurs whenever the sampling frequency is less than twice the highest frequency component of signal frequency, according to the Nyquist theorem [12].

EMG recording is usually done at a maximum frequency of 500 Hz, and the sample should be at least 1000 Hz. To analyze muscle activity in the most comprehensive way possible, it is advisable to work with a sampling rate on the order of 2000 Hz, with the highest frequency component of the signal always limited by the low-pass filter [4, 12, 28].

## 8.3. Calibration

The measured physical magnitude is converted to voltage using a sensor or transducer, which is then applied to the A/D converter. Knowing the input range and resolution of the A/D converter, one can calculate the voltage of the converter input value from the digitized value, as shown in Figure 8.

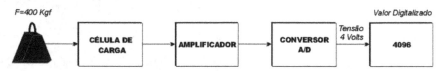

**Figure 8.** Relationship of physical quantity to a digital signal [3].

## 9. Mathematical processing

Two types of processing are usually used in research: time domain processing, used when one is interested in the temporal analysis of EMG amplitude, and frequency domain processing [1, 26, 28].

### 9.1. Processing in the time domain

In order to process EMG signals in the time domain, there is a set of processing procedures for characterizing the curve and measuring the signal strength during muscle contraction. Having several kinesiological applications, EMG time domain analysis is often used in areas such as neuromuscular coordination, motor control, the relationship between EMG and muscle force or human movement [25].

*9.1.1. Removing the slow-drift (or DC) component present in the signal*

Sometimes the signal involves a DC component that causes displacement of the baseline signal. This component is a common signal that has no relation with myoelectric activity. It can be the result of electrochemical phenomena between the electrodes and skin or the limitations of the amplifiers. An easy way to remove it is to calculate the average of all sampling points and shift the curve of the EMG result (high-pass filter) [12, 28].

## 9.1.2. Signal rectification

Correcting the curve is an operation normally used to enable the subsequent integration of the signal, since it transforms a curve containing both positive and negative values (Figure 10) and a zero mean to a curve of only positive absolute values (Figure 11).

There are two ways to rectify the curve: eliminating the negative values (half-wave rectification), or reversing the negative values and adding them to the positive values (full wave rectification). Full-wave rectification has the advantage of maintaining all of the information contained in the signal, unlike half-wave rectification [5, 28].

## 9.1.3. Root-mean-square value of the signal

The RMS is the amount of continuous signal able to contain the same amount of energy. It is mathematically defined as the square root of the mean of the squares of the instantaneous values of the signal [4, 12, 22, 23].

## 9.1.4. Normalization of the signal in the time domain

One problem when comparing different EMG signals has to do with differences in the duration of the various signals to be compared.

Normalizing means transforming, without changing the signal's structure, the duration differences into signals with the same number of samples. This can be done, for example, by taking the signal containing the lowest number of samples as a reference. An algorithm can be applied that determines, depending on the duration of each signal, the number of samples to be removed at certain intervals, reducing all signals to the same number of samples contained in the shorter of the two signals, and thus retaining the original forms [16].

## 9.1.5. Amplitude normalization

The EMG signal varies greatly upon comparison with recordings from the same individual or different individuals. The absolute value of the EMG signal thus provides little information, especially when dealing with signals from different individuals or the same individual at different times. One way to compensate for this limitation is to normaliz EMG amplitude curves. This technique consists of transforming the absolute amplitude values of the different curves to be compared into values relative to a reference EMG taken as 100% [4, 7, 15].

## 9.1.6. Integral of the EMG signal

The mathematical interpretation of the integral concept consists of determining the area enclosed by curve, whether an EMG or any other signal. In the case of the EMG, so that the result of integration is not zero, a rectified signal must be used. By integrating the EMG signal, a result that is proportional to the number of electrical impulses is obtained [3].

### 9.1.7. Filtering of the rectified signal

The signals collected in real time in the original format are stored in files. After this phase certain mathematical processes are applied. The purpose of this processing is to make correction, i.e., to transform negative signals into positive signals. This is necessary to allow averaging of the analyzed signal, since if such correction is not performed, the average of the signals will be near zero. This is because the negative and positive are symmetrical. In the post-rectification, a 5 Hz low-pass filter can be run in order to have a signal wrap. The lower the value of this filter, the smoother the curve will be [27, 28].

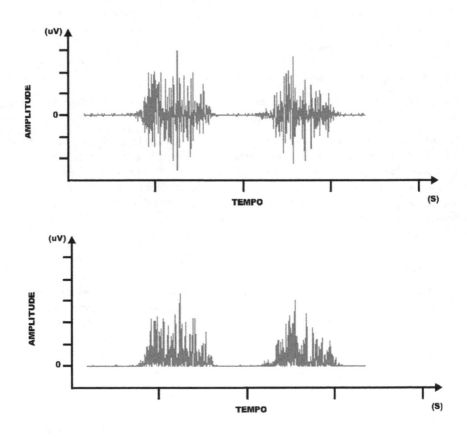

**Figure 9.** A) original signal interference. B) rectified original signal [3].

### 9.2. Processing the frequency domain – Spectral analysis

The EMG signal's frequencies are distributed between 1 and 500 Hz, with a great concentration between 20 and 250 Hz in the case of simple muscular activity. The distribution of energy at different frequencies (power spectral density) reflects the predominance of the low or high frequency components in the signal and has been used in kinesiological research. Factors that influence the spectral profile of the EMG signal have been listed by various authors.

EMG can be considered an overlapping of the action potentials of all the active motor units. The spectrum of EMG frequencies thus contains information about the characteristics of different fibers that contribute to the signal. Spectral analysis can provide information about the mean duration of the active fiber potentials, which in turn can be used to determine the mean velocity of muscle fiber conduction [3,4].

## 10. Conclusion

For dynamic sampling, active electrodes (with preamps) are less susceptible to artifacts or ambient noise, which can be observed when comparing them with signals collected during isometric contractions in volunteers with dysfunctions.

EMG signals are affected by the anatomical and physiological properties of muscles, the peripheral nervous system and the instrumentation used to collect the signal. Thus it is important to understand basic muscle functions to correctly record EMG signals [12].

It can be said that signal processing begins, indirectly, as soon as the electrodes are placed. Electrode placement involves several factors that are decisive for the level and purity of the EMG signal to be collected, including: cleaning the skin, the amount and temperature of the conductive gel, the position of the electrodes and the signal-to-noise ratio, which expresses the balance between the energy of the signal generated during muscle contraction and the energy of noise from various undesirable sources [27].

Therefore, sEMG can be recommended as a tool for analyzing and interpreting electrical signals emanated during muscular contractions in both normal and pathological situations and can be applied in the study of motor function and functional rehabilitation [4].

## 11. Future directions

Studies in the field of signal processing, especially, surface electromyography signals, have been widely used for understanding the dynamic motions by the fact that most human movements happening dynamically. Thus, processing in the field of time and frequency should be increasingly directed to this specificity.

Understanding the phenomena of depolarization of motor units, future research should be related to the physiological, mechanophysiological and functional human movement.

Applications in the area of functional biomechanics, ergonomics, rehabilitation, sports and physical activity must be analyzed dynamically so that the signal processing, fairly represent the specific characteristics of human movement-environment relationship. Thus, these factors provide parameters for understanding the non-stationary signals, the variation components of the muscle fiber in relation to the positioning of the electrodes and in the bioelectrical conductivity.

## Author details

César Ferreira Amorim
*University of City of São Paulo- UNICID, São Paulo - SP, Brazil*

Runer Augusto Marson
*Sports Center, Federal University of Ouro Preto, Ouro Preto - MG, Brazil*

## 12. References

[1]  Acierno, S.P. Baratta, R.V., Solomonow, M. A pratical guide to electromyography for biomechanists. Lousiana: State University, 1995.

[2]  Amadio, A.C. ; Duarte, M. Fundamentos Biomecânicos para análise do movimento. São Paulo: Editora Laboratório de Biomecânica EEFUSP, 162p. 1996.

[3]  Amorim, C.F; Hirata,Tamotsu. Behavior analysis of electromyographic activity of the masseter muscle in sleep bruxers, Journal of Bodywork & Movement Therapies (2009), doi:10.1016/j.jbmt.2008.12.002

[4]  Amorim, C.F. Sistema de Aquisição de Sinais Eletromiográficos com Eletrodos Bipolares com Pré-Amplificação. In: 3c Biomédica,18., Setembro de 2002. Anais... São José dos Campos: Univap, 2002.

[5]  Andrade, A.D.; Silva,T.N.S.;Vasconcelos, H.; Marcelino, M.; Rodrigues-Machado, M.G.; Filho, G.; Moraes, M.; Marinho, P.E.M.; Amorim, C.F. Inspiratory muscular activation during threshold therapy in elderly healthy and patients with COPD, Journal of Electromyography and Kinesiology (2005), doi:10.1016/j.jelekin.2005.06.002

[6]  Araujo, R.C.;Amadio, A .C.; Furlani, J. Contribuição para a interpretação da relação força e atividade EMG. In: Congresso Nacional De Biomecânica, 4.,1992, São Paulo. Anais... São Paulo: Escola de Educação Física da Universidade de São Paulo, 1992. p. 146-153.

[7]  Araujo, R.C.; Duarte, M.; Amadio, A .C. Evaluation of increase in force and EMG Activity´s Cirves. In: Congress Of The International Society Of Biomechanics, 15., Jyvaskyla, 1995. Abstract... Jyvaskyla, University Of Jyvaskyla, 1995. p.64-65.

[8]  Baba, K.; Akishige, S.; Yaka, T.; Ai, M. Influence of alteration of occlusal relationship on activity of jaw closing muscles and mandibular movement during submaximal clenching. Journal of Oral Rehabilitation. v.27, p.783-801.2000.

[9] Bardsley, P.A., Bentley, S., Hall, H.S., Singh, S.J., Evans, D.H., Morgan, M.D., 1993. Measurement of inspiratory muscle performance with incremental threshold loading: a comparison of two techniques. Thorax 48, 354-359.

[10] Basmajian, J.V. Muscle Alive. 4 ed. Baltimore: Willians & Wilkins, 1978.

[11] Basmajian, J.V. Muscles alive: their function revealed by electromyography. Baltimore: Williams e Wilkins, 1962.

[12] Basmajian, J.V.; De Luca, C.J. Muscle alive: their function revealed by electromyography. 5a ed. Baltimore, Williams e Wiikins, 1985. p.501-561

[13] Biasotto, D. A. Estudo eletromiográfico de músculos do sistema estomatognático durante a mastigação de diferentes materiais. Dissertação(Mestrado) - Faculdade de Odontolocia de Piracicaba da UNICAMP, 2000. 134p.

[14] Blanksma, N.G ;Van Eijden, T.M.G.J. Electromyographic Heterogeneity in the Humam Temporalis and Masseter Muscles during Static Biting. Open Close Excursion, and Chewi. Journal of Dental Research. v.74, n.6,p. 1318- 1327. June 1995.

[15] Dainty, D.A.; Norman, R.W. Standarding biomechanical testing in sport. Champaign, Human Kinetics, 1987.

[16] Ervilha, U.F., Duarte, M Amadio, A.C. Estudo sobre procedimento de normalização do sinal eletromiográfico durante o movimento humano. Rev. Bras. Fisiot., p.15-20,1998

[17] Hatze, H. The meaning of the term"Biomechanics". Journal of Biomechanics, v.7,p.189-190,1974.

[18] Landulpho, A.B. et al. The effect of the oclusal splints on the treatment of temporomandibular disorders – a computerized electromyographic study of masseter and anterior temporalis muscles. Electomyogr. Clin. Neurophysiol. v.42, p.187-191.2002.

[19] M.A. Mananas, R. Jane, J.A. Fiz, J. Morera, P. Caminal, Study of myographic signals from sternomastoid muscle in patients with chronics obstructive pulmonary disease, IEEE Trans. Biomed. Eng. V.47, p. 674-681. 2000.

[20] Mclean L. The effect of postural correction on muscle activation amplitudes recorded from the cervicobrachial region. J Electromyogr Kinesiol., v.15,p.527–535. 2005.

[21] Nascimento, L.N.; Amorim, C.F.; Giannasi, L.C.; Oliveira, C.S.;Nacif, S.R.; Silva, A.M.; Nascimento,D.F.F.; Marchini, Daniela; Oliveira,L.V.F., Occlusal splint for sleep bruxism: na electromyographic associated to Helkimo Index evoluation, Sleep Breath,v.12, p.275–280, 2008.DOI 10.1007/s11325-007-0152-8

[22] Nobre, M.E.P.N.; Lopes, F.; Cordeiro, L.; Marinho, P.E.M.; Silva, T.N.S.S.; Amorim, C.F.; Cahalin, L.P.; Andrade, A.D., Inspiratory muscle endurance testing: pulmonary ventilation and electromyographic analysis, Respiratory Physiology & Neurobiology, (2006), doi:10.1016/j.resp.2006.04.005

[23] Politti, F., Amorim C.F., Calili L., Andrade, A.O., Palomari, E.T., The use of surface electromyography for the study of auricular acupuncture, Journal of Bodywork & Movement Therapies (2009), doi:10.1016/j.jbmt.2008.11.006

[24] Portney, L. Eletromiografia e testes de velocidade de condução nervosa. In: O'sullivan, S.B.; Schmitz, T.J. Fisioterapia: avaliação e tratamento. 2 ed. São Paulo- Manole, 1993. Cap. 10, p. 183-223.

[25] Soderberg, G.L. & Cook, T.M. Electromyography in Biomechanics. Physical Therapy, v.64, p.: 1813-20,1984.

[26] Suda, E.Y; Amorim, C.F.; Sacco, I.C.N. Influence of ankle functional instability on the ankle electromyography during landin after volleyball blocking, Journal of Electromyography and Kinesiology (2007), doi:10.1016/j.jelekin.2007.10.007

[27] Turker, K.S. Electromyographyc: Some methodological problems and issues. Physical .Therapy. v.73, n.10,p. 698-710, 1993.

[28] Winter, D.A. Biomechanics and Motor Control of Human Movement. New York: John Wiley & Sons Inc.,1990.

# Chapter 9

# Proposal of a Neuro Fuzzy System for Myoelectric Signal Analysis from Hand-Arm Segment

Gabriela Winkler Favieiro and Alexandre Balbinot

Additional information is available at the end of the chapter

## 1. Introduction

Many with disabilities have some difficulties in integrating into society due to impossibility or to restriction in performing simple tasks of day-to-day. This situation is gradually changing by virtue of technological development in the biomedical instrumentation area in respect of human rehabilitation and especially with in the development of assistive technology managed by computational intelligence (computing algorithms and learning machines using techniques as fuzzy logic, artificial neural networks, genetic algorithms, support vector machines, among others). Scientific researches in this area are allowing the development of several mechanisms to improve the life quality of people with special needs, making them more independent and more likely to real social and economical integration.

It's possible to cite, for example, research related to robotic prosthesis. The development of system managed by myoelectric signals (MES) with the intention to mimic the human arm movement, is far from perfect, making the subject of many researches (Ajiboye & Weir, 2005; Chan et al., 2000; Englehart & Hudgins, 2003; Favieiro & Balbinot, 2011; Favieiro et al., 2011; Hincapie & Kirsch, 2009; Hudgins et al., 1991; Hudgins et al., 1994; Jacobsen et al., 1982; Katutoshi et al., 1992; Khushaba et al., 2010; Momen et al., 2007; Park & Meek, 1995). These researches are mainly being conducted in able-bodies subjects to verify the feasibility and performance of different algorithms for pattern recognition using EMG signals from the forearm muscles. In these studies are usually employed a high number of electrode pairs, ranging from 4 to 12. Using classification patterns techniques such as LDA, fuzzy logic, among others, was found high accuracies (>90%) for the classification of different moves ranging from four to ten. Develop a robotic prosthesis as similar as possible to the human arm is not a simple task. There are great difficulties both in the area of distinguish the various degrees of freedom that the arm can have as developing a robotic prosthesis that can accomplish or replicate all these movements.

Briefly, the myoelectric signal is the bio-signal muscle control of the human body which contains the information of the user's intent to contract a muscle and, therefore, perform a certain movement. Studies have shown that amputees are able to repeatedly generate certain standard myoelectric signals in front of intention to carry out a particular movement. It makes the use of such signal highly advantageous, because the control of a robotic prosthesis can be accomplished according to user's intention to perform a specified movement. Furthermore, detection of the myoelectric signal can be obtained noninvasively through surface electrodes. Although the distress signal has low amplitude (mV range) is sufficient for its analysis and surface electrodes are far more hygienic and convenient as the removal, insertion and sterilization can be accomplished by the user.

Therefore, it is possible to distinguish certain muscle movements while processing the electrical parameters of the myoelectric signal both in time domain and frequency domain. With the characterized movements is possible to control a robotic prosthesis that aims to replicate, the best possible, the movements of a human arm. Considering that premise, this research aims to study and develop a system that uses myoelectric signals, acquired by surface electrodes, to characterize certain movements of the human arm, allowing studies between man and machine with adequate precision for future enabling the actual replacement of an amputee limb with a robotic prosthesis suitable and intuitively controlled through the remaining muscle signals. To recognize certain hand-arm segment movements, was developed an algorithm for pattern recognition technique based on neuro-*fuzzy*, representing the core of this research. This algorithm has as input the preprocessed myoelectric signal, to disclosed specific characteristics of the signal, and as output the performed movement.

The present research was also preoccupy in not only distinguish certain simple movements of the human arm, but also characterize complex movements that combine several degrees of freedom, making this study more closely to the reality, in which more degrees of freedom represents an improve in the life quality of people with special needs, making them more likely to real integration in the society.

## 2. Soft computing

The understanding, processing or solving complex problems require intelligent systems that combine knowledge, techniques and methodologies from various sources (Zadeh, 1992). Thus, intelligent systems should aggregate human knowledge in a specific domain, adapt and learn the best way possible in environments that are constantly changing. For this reasons, it is very advantageous to use several computational techniques instead of just one, which is the essence of neuro-*fuzzy* technique: neural networks that recognize patterns and are able to adapt to changes and the *fuzzy* inference system that incorporates human knowledge for making decisions.

Typically a fuzzy system incorporates a rule base, membership functions and an inference procedure and has been presenting success in systems with applications in the presence of ambiguous elements (Begg et al., 2008; Zadeh et al., 2004). Systems combining neural networks with fuzzy systems usually have the following characteristics (Jang, 1997):

- human knowledge presented in the form of rules, for example, if-then;
- computational models based on biological models, such as the use of neural networks for pattern recognition;
- optimization techniques, such as the use of a hybrid technique;
- construction of a model with data sample;
- numerical computation instead of symbolic computation.

This chapter briefly presents the fuzzy techniques, adaptive algorithms, neuro-fuzzy and data clustering used in the present research.

## 2.1. Fuzzy logic

A fuzzy set is defined as a set or collection of elements with membership values between 0 and 1. Therefore, the transition between belonging or not belonging to the set is gradual and is characterized by its fuzzy Membership Function (MF) that is used to describe the fuzzy membership value given to fuzzy set elements (Begg et al., 2008) enabling the fuzzy set model linguist expression used in everyday life, such as, "the rms value of the masseter myoelectric signal is medium high". For these reasons, the fuzzy sets theory is very efficient when dealing with concepts of ambiguity (Zadeh, 1992) and allows its use in several applications.

Therefore, a fuzzy set not-empty $Z$ in a given space $X$ ($Z \subseteq X$), is the set represented by equations (1) e (2):

$$Z = \{(x, \mu_Z(x)); x \epsilon X\} \tag{1}$$

$$\mu_Z: X \rightarrow [0,1] \tag{2}$$

since $\mu_Z$ a membership function of an specified fuzzy set. This function indicates for each element $x \epsilon X$ its membership degree to the fuzzy set $Z$ between three possibilities (Rutkowski, 2005):

- $\mu_Z(x) = 1$ means the full membership of element $x$ to the fuzzy set $Z$, in others words, $x \epsilon Z$;
- $\mu_Z(x) = 0$ means the lack of membership of element $x$ to the fuzzy set $Z$, in others words, $x \notin Z$;
- $0 < \mu_Z(x) < 1$ means a partial membership of element $x$ to the fuzzy set $Z$.

### 2.1.1. Standard forms of membership functions

A membership function (MF) is a curve that defines how a point in the input space is mapped into a membership degree between 0 and 1 (Dubois, 1980). Typically a MF is defined by a mathematical expression. Following is a few membership functions ($\mu_Z(x)$) commonly used.

The triangular membership function or simply membership function of class $t$ is defined by equation (3):

$$\mu_Z(x) = t(x; a, b, c) = \begin{cases} 0, & x \leq a \\ \frac{x-a}{b-a}, & a \leq x \leq b \\ \frac{c-x}{c-b}, & b \leq x \leq c \\ 0, & c \leq x \end{cases} \tag{3}$$

where $b$ is the modal value ($a < b < c$) and $a$ and $b$ are the upper and lower bounds of $t(x;a,b,c)$, respectively.

The Gaussian-membership function é specified by equation (4):

$$\mu_Z(x) = g(x; \sigma) = exp\left(-\left(\frac{x-\bar{x}}{\sigma}\right)^2\right) \tag{4}$$

where $\bar{x}$ is the middle and $\sigma$ defines the width of the Gaussian curve. It is the most common membership function (Rutkowski, 2005). While Bell membership function é specified by equation (5):

$$\mu_Z(x) = bell(x; a, b, c) = \frac{1}{1+\left|\frac{x-c}{a}\right|^{2b}} \tag{5}$$

where the parameter $a$ defines its width, the parameter $b$ its slopes, and the parameter $c$ its center.

Other membership functions found in some applications are $\Gamma$-membership function, $S$-membership function, trapezoidal-membership function and exponential-membership functions. For more details, see (Rutkowski, 2005). As an example, Figure 1 shows the standard format of the MF Gaussian and MF Bell.

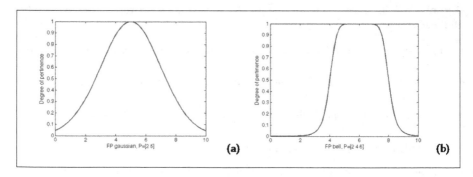

**Figure 1.** Membership function: (a) Gaussian and (b) bell.

The triangle and trapezoidal function are widely used in several applications because they are simple expressions and have suitable computational efficiency for real-time applications. However, these two membership functions are composed of straight line segments showing no soft edge at their ends. As a result, the Gaussian and Bell membership functions are increasingly used to specify fuzzy sets (Jang, 1997).

### 2.1.2. Fuzzy reasoning and Sugeno fuzzy inference system

In general, the fuzzy reasoning process can be divided into four main steps that are used in a fuzzy inference system (Dubois, 1980):

- comparison of the known facts to the fuzzy rules background facts to determine the compatibility degree for each of the antecedent membership function;
- combination of compatibility degrees in relation to the antecedents membership functions in a rule using fuzzy operators, for example, 'AND' or 'OR' to form the firing strength that indicates the degree whose part of the antecedent rule is satisfied;
- application of firing strength for the consequent membership function of a rule to generate a qualified consequent membership function that represents how the firing strength was propagated and utilized in a fuzzy implication statement;
- selection of all qualified consequent membership functions for the general output membership.

A fuzzy set is characterized by its membership function and operations on fuzzy sets manipulate these functions. For further details on fuzzy operations such as adding, subtracting, inverse operation, scaling operation, among others, just as, fuzzy relations and their properties consult the works indicated in the references of this chapter (Begg et al., 2008; Dubois, 1980; Rutkowski, 2005).

In recent years, different structures of neuro-fuzzy networks have been proposed combining the advantages of neural networks and fuzzy logic (Rutkowski, 2005). Several studies using the Mamdani type interference or the Takagi-Sugeno model. For this study the Sugeno fuzzy model proposed by Takagi, Sugeno and Kang (Sugeno, 1988; Takagi, 1985) had been used to generate fuzzy rules from a set of input and outputs. A typical fuzzy rule in the Sugeno fuzzy model is shown in (6):

$$\text{If } x \text{ is equal to A and } y \text{ is equal to B, then } z=f(x,y) \tag{6}$$

as A and B sets of fuzzy antecedents and $z= f(x,y)$ the crisp consecutive function. Considering the computational performance and the mathematical operations usually used (for instance, weighted sum) the Sugeno fuzzy model is the most popular inference system for fuzzy modeling based on input data (Jang, 1993)

## 2.2. Adaptive Neuro Fuzzy Inference System

Adaptive Neuro Fuzzy Inference System or ANFIS is a class of adaptive networks whose functionality is equivalent to a fuzzy inference system, proposed by Jang, which generates a fuzzy rule base and membership functions automatically (Jang, 1993).

Typically the ANFIS network topology consists of connected nodes that depend on parameters that change according to certain learning rules that minimize the error criteria. The learning technique most commonly used is the gradient method, however Jang proposed hybrid learning rule which includes the Least Square or simply LSE Estimator (Jang, 1993).

Considering a fuzzy system with three inputs x, y and z one output, v and a fuzzy inference Sugeno model. One possible set of rules is shown in equations (7) and (8):

Rule 1: If x is equal to $A_1$, y is equal to $B_1$, and z is equal to $C_1$, then $f_1 = p_1x + q_1y + r_1y + s_1$ (7)

Rule 2: If x is equal to $A_2$, y is equal to $B_2$, and z is equal to $C_2$, then $f_2 = p_2x + q_2y + r_2z + s_2$ (8)

as an example, Figure 2 illustrates the reasoning mechanism for the Sugeno inference model. The equivalent ANFIS architecture is presented in Figure 3 with nodes of same layer having similar functions. Following is an explanation for each of the network layers based on Jang's excellent text (Jang, 1997).

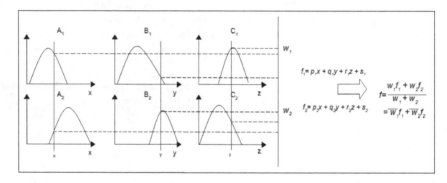

**Figure 2.** Example of a Sugeno inference model containing three inputs and two rules.

The first layer of Figure 3 is represented by adaptive nodes $i$ whose functions are determined by equations (9), (10) and (11):

$$O_{1,i} = \mu_{A_i}(x), \quad para\ i = 1, 2 \tag{9}$$

$$O_{1,i} = \mu_{B_{i-2}}(y), \quad para\ i = 3, 4 \tag{10}$$

$$O_{1,i} = \mu_{C_{i-4}}(y), \quad para\ i = 5, 6 \tag{11}$$

where x, y or z entries in node $i$ and $A_i$ $B_{i-2}$ and $C_{i-4}$ linguistic labels associated with that node. Thus, $O_{1,i}$ represents the pertinence degree to the fuzzy set A ($A_1$, $A_2$, $B_1$, $B_2$, $C_1$ or $C_2$) and specifies the degree to each input x, y or z satisfies the fuzzy set A. The membership function $\mu$ can be any of the membership functions presented in section 2.1.1. Importantly, when the values (called the premise parameters) of the membership function are changed, the function varies, i.e., display various types of MF to the fuzzy set A.

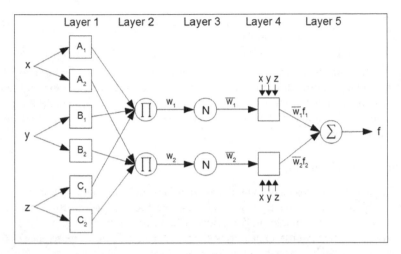

**Figure 3.** The equivalent ANFIS architecture of the Sugeno Fuzzy model represented in Figure 2.

The layer 2 has fixed nodes indicated by $\Pi$ with outputs that represents the input signals product, as indicated in equation (12) – the output nodes represent the firing strength of a given rule:

$$O_{2,1} = \omega_i = \mu_{A_i}(x)\mu_{B_i}(y)\mu_{C_i}(z), \quad i = 1, 2. \tag{12}$$

In layer 3 the fixed nodes are referred to $N$. The $i_{th}$ node calculates the firing strength rate of rule $i_{th}$ to the sum of all firing strength of rules, given by equation (13) – the nodes in layer 3 are generally known as normalized firing strength:

$$O_{3,i} = \overline{\omega_i} = \frac{\omega_i}{\omega_1 + \omega_2}, \quad i = 1, 2. \tag{13}$$

Layer 4, for example, the nodes $i$ are adaptive with the function given by equation (14):

$$O_{4,i} = \overline{\omega_i}f_i = \overline{\omega_i}(p_i x + q_i y + r_i z + s_i), \tag{14}$$

where $\overline{\omega_i}$ is a normalized firing strength from layer 3 and $\{p_i, q_i, r_i, s_i\}$ the set of parameters (called consequence parameters) of this node.

The last layer of the Figure 3 has only one fixed node called $\Sigma$ that determines the final output as the sum of all signals represented by equation (15):

$$final\ output = O_{5,1} = \sum_i \overline{\omega_i}f_i = \frac{\sum_i \omega_i f_i}{\sum_i \omega_i} \tag{15}$$

Considering the architecture shown in Figure 3 it can be seen that while the values of the parameters of the premises is fixed, the final output can be expressed as a linear combination of consequence parameters. Therefore, the output can be rewritten, for example, by the linear equation with the following consequence parameters: $p_1$, $q_1$, $r_1$, $s_1$, $p_2$, $q_2$, $r_2$ and $s_2$ (see equation 16):

$$f \begin{array}{l} = \\ = \\ = \end{array} \begin{array}{l} \frac{\omega_1}{\omega_1+\omega_2}f_1 + \frac{\omega_2}{\omega_1+\omega_2}f_2 \\ \overline{\omega_i}(p_1 x + q_1 y + r_1 z + s_1) + \overline{\omega_2}(p_2 x + q_2 y + r_2 z + s_2) \\ (\overline{\omega_i}x)p_1 + (\overline{\omega_i}y)q_1 + (\overline{\omega_i}z)r_1 + (\overline{\omega_i})s_1 + (\overline{\omega_2}x)p_2 + (\overline{\omega_2}y)q_2 + (\overline{\omega_2}z)r_2 + (\overline{\omega_2})s_2 \end{array} \qquad (16)$$

The hybrid training algorithm is based on the following criteria: In the forward step of the hybrid algorithm, the outputs of the nodes will forward to the layer 4 and the consequence parameters are identified by the least squares method. In the backward step, the error signal is propagated backward and the premise parameters are updated by gradient descent method (Jang, 1993)

## 2.3. Subtractive clustering

The utilization of clustering algorithms allows characterization and organization of data, but also the construction of models from a database. Basically clustering divides data sets derived from a large group into similar groups. Clustering can be used to model an initial fuzzy network, in other words, to determine the fuzzy rules. For this purpose, the clustering technique is validated based on the following propositions:

- Similar entries in a target system should be modeled to produce similar outputs;
- These similar pairs input-output are packed in clusters of the training data set.

The technique subtractive clustering proposed by Chiu, considers any data points as candidates for the cluster centers (Chiu, 1994). Using this method, the processing is proportional to the number of data points, independent of the size of the problem under consideration.

For example, is a collection of n data points {x1,...,xn} in an M-dimensional space, whose points were normalized to a hypercube. Since each data point is candidate for the cluster center, the density measurement at each point xi is defined by equation (17):

$$D_i = \sum_{j=1}^{n} \exp\left(-\frac{\|x_i - x_j\|^2}{(r_a/2)^2}\right) \qquad (17)$$

where $r_a$ is a positive constant. A point will have a great density it has many neighbor points. The radius $r_a$ defines the neighborhood and the points outside of the neighborhood contribute very little to the density measurement.

After the density measurement ($D_i$) is calculated for all of the points, the point with highest density is selected to be the center of the first cluster. If $x_{c1}$ is the selected point and $D_{c1}$ your density value, the measured density for each point is revised according to the expression shown in (18):

$$D_i = D_i - D_{c1}\exp\left(-\frac{\|x_i - x_{c1}\|^2}{(r_b/2)^2}\right) \qquad (18)$$

After reviewing the density of each point, the next center $x_{c2}$ is selected and all of the density measures of the points are revised again. This process is repeated until a sufficient number of clusters are created. When applied the *subtractive clustering* technique for a set of input-output data, each cluster center will represents a prototype that exhibits certain characteristics of the system being modeled. This cluster centers are used as centers of the premises of the fuzzy rules in a zero order Sugeno model.

## 3. Experimental methods

To help understanding, a block diagram of the proposed system is presented in the Figure 4. In the following sections are presented detailed discussions of the key elements that make up this block diagram.

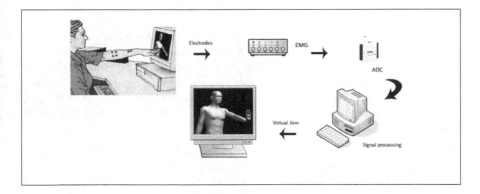

**Figure 4.** Block diagram of the purposed system.

The proposed experimental apparatus consists of an LCD screen that generates visual stimulus with animations of random movements of the hand-arm segment which should be replicated by the user An 8-channel electromyography is used with surface electrodes placed in strategic places and previously defined in the right arm to capture the myoelectric signal during displayed movements. Through a data acquisition board, the myoelectric signal is digitized and processed in a portable computer, where it is filtered and analyzed by software using the technique of pattern recognition, based on neuro fuzzy systems. Finally, the system has as output the characterization of the movement and also verifies if the executed movement was well recognized.

### 3.1. Electromyograph and data acquisition system

Electromyograph is a device used to capture the myoelectric signals with the help of electrodes. The electromyograph used in this work was developed in the research project coordinated by Balbinot (Balbinot, 2005).

The recording signal is performed using bipolar electrodes of passive configuration. Located near the electrodes, in each acquisition cable, was used an instrumentation amplifier with differential input, INA118, to minimize the noise as the amplitude of the acquired signal is in mV. The signal is amplified up to 1000 times

The frequency of the muscular signals captured by the surface electrodes has a range varying from 20 to 500 Hz. Due to this fact, the EMG designed consist of two cascaded second order low-pass filters with a cutoff frequency at 1000 Hz, and two cascaded second order high-pass filters with cutoff frequency at 20Hz.

To perform the data acquisition was chosen the National Instruments acquisition board NI USB 6008. This board features eight analog input channels with 10 bit resolution and sampling rate of 10 kS/s. In this study we used the eight analog input channels (one entry per channel) with an acquisition rate of 1 kHz per channel.

## 3.2. Virtual model

Virtual human body models are used in many applications that allow human-machine Interaction. The virtual model created in this work aims to help the standardization of tests for the acquisition of the myoelectric signal. With this virtual model is possible, for the Subject, visualize the movement to be performed during the tests, so that all Subjects perform as best as possible, the same movements at the same time base and at the same time, leaving the system more user-friendly. For the development of the virtual model we used the software MakeHuman Alpha5 and Blender 1.0 Beta 2:54.

Initially, MakeHuman software was used to define the parameters of the humanoid (height, weight, sex) that is subsequently exported to the software Blender. This virtual model is a skeleton whose manipulative joints are used to define the positions that it should take (Tale & Balbinot, 2011). For the development of the animation it was necessary to set the start and end position and movement timing of each of the respective movement. The software then builds an animation by connecting the two points during a defined duration. Also was established a rest position which was adopted for all movements. Importantly, all movements start from the rest position, run and return to it. It should be noted that after the generation of virtual models, a video of the animations are created using a standard rate of 24 fps Avi format.

To display the animations, a routine in Labview was developed enabling the reading of Avi files and reproduction of videos representing the virtual model through a window of Windows Media Player. This window opens in the auxiliary display (LCD screen in Figure 4) being viewed only by the user of the system. The operator sees only the Labview programming window on the laptop screen, where it is shown that the signal is being acquired during the tests.

The set of movements generated through the virtual model was divided into two groups: simple and complex movements (sequence of simple movements). There are seven simple movements represented in Figure 5, which are: wrist flexion; hand contraction, wrist extension, forearm flexion, forearm rotation, hand adduction and hand abduction. For the simple movements were adopted the following time sequence with a total duration of each animation of 8.3 s:

• Initial interval: 0,4 s in which the animation will be on rest position;

- forward movement: duration of 2,9 s;
- movement interval: 1,25 s, in which the animation keeps static at the end the going movement;
- backward movement: same duration of the forward movement (2,9 s);
- final interval: duration of 0,8 s, which the animation is again on rest position; .

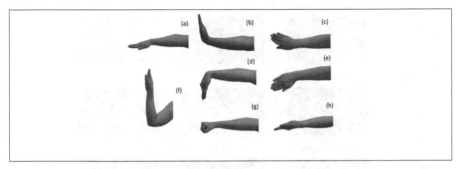

**Figure 5.** Pictures representing the simple movements created by the virtual model: (a) resting position, (b) wrist extension, (c) wrist adduction, (d) wrist flexion (e) wrist abduction, (f) forearm flexion, (g) hand contraction and (h) forearm rotation.

In the Figure 6 is shown a static representation of the simple movements presented in video format.

The movements that are called complex are characterized by a combination of determined basic movements defined above. For this study, five complex movements were selected as shown in Figure 7, that are: hand contraction with forearm rotation, forearm rotation with forearm flexion; forearm rotation with forearm flexion and wrist flexion, hand contraction with forearm flexion and wrist extension and flexion.

For the animations of the complex movements, the same parameters of the simple movement animations were been used, but with total duration of 17 second for each complex movement.

## 3.3. Experimental procedures

All the experiments were carried out with consent of the Subjects, according to the ethical precepts and respecting the bio signal acquisition techniques (in this case related to the myoelectric signal acquisition), like for instance the treatment of the skin, electrode positioning among other aspects.

For the data acquisition the NI USB 6008 board was used. Eight pairs of electrodes located in the main muscle groups of the Subject were been used, which are the main part of the movements that were chosen to characterize: Biceps (C0), palmaris longus (C1), flexor carpi ulnaris (C2), flexor carpi radialis (C3), pronator teres (C4), extensor digitorum (C5), brachioradialis (C6) and extensor carpi ulnaris (C7), as shown in Figure 8.

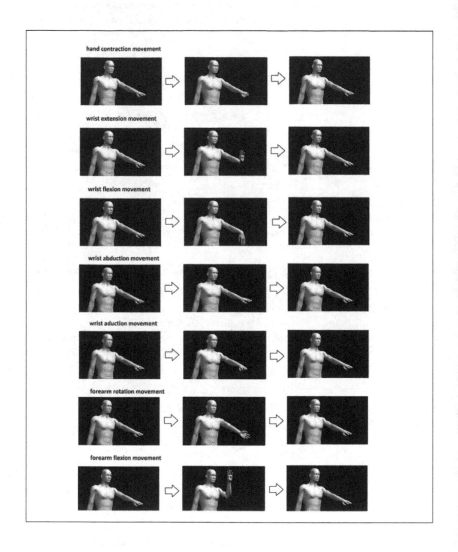

**Figure 6.** Diagram representing the videos of simple movements developed as a virtual model.

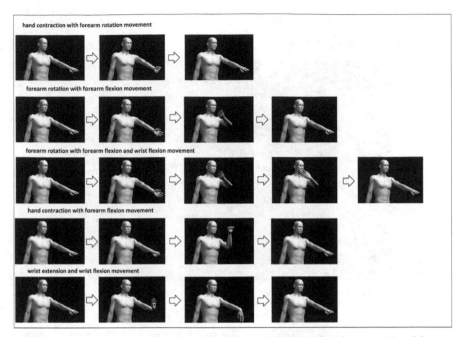

**Figure 7.** Diagram representing the videos of complex movements developed as a virtual model.

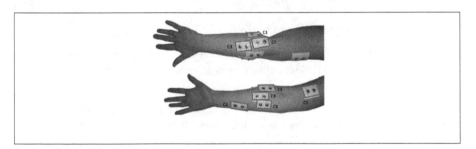

**Figure 8.** Picture showing the electrodes positions.

To start the acquisition, after correct positioning of the electrodes, the Subject is instructed to replicate the animations of the virtual model, which appear on the LCD screen, using a moderate strength. In order to standardize the testing of signal acquisition was adapted to the methodology proposed by Li (Li, 2010), considering the following aspects:

- each test consists of 5 sessions;
- is generated a random sequence of animations for each session of the test;
- each session is composed of 5 repetitions of each of the 12 selected movements;
- between movements, the Subject should rest for 3 seconds;

- each Subject participates in a single test.

In the figure 9 is shown a picture of one of the sessions.

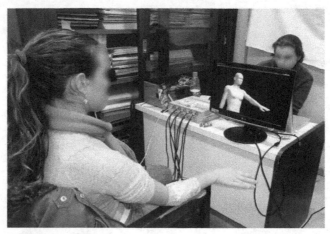

**Figure 9.** Picture of a session.

A Labview routine was developed to interface with Matlab to generate the sequence of movements (See figures 6 and 7) randomly. The output is a vector with a random order of the movements of the virtual model presented to the user.

### 3.4. Acquisition and signal pre processing

The programming language chosen for the development of the proposed system software is Labview (Laboratory Virtual Instrument Engineering Workbench) from National Instruments.

The acquisition and generation of the myoelectric signals database were obtained through a routine created in Labview software to read the input data acquired through the NI USB 6008 card and store them in a file.

To choose the sample rate was considered that the myoelectric signal of interest in this work is in the range 20-500 Hz, and most of the energy of this signal is in the frequency range 50-150 Hz based on this information, the sampling frequency used was 1 kHz which is suitable for the proposed system. For this specification, 1 ms was sufficient to identify the user movements.

The online acquisition is performed in a way that the signal is transferred to the computer in time windows of 50 ms, thought the acquisition board, and the signal is stored in a FIFO (First In First Out) queue, in which the stored time windows are being processed according to the acquisition order, ensuring no data loss. Figure 10 shows the corresponding flowchart of this stage.

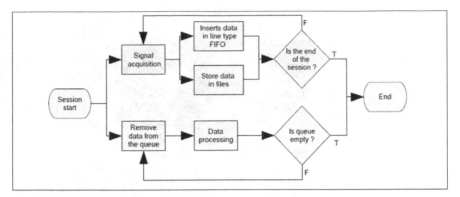

**Figure 10.** Flowchart of the online acquisition routine.

According to the flowchart shown in Figure 10, the data acquisition and processing are used simultaneously, since it is possible to perform parallel routines in Labview (note that the real parallelism is only supported from the Labview 2010 package).

### 3.4.1. Calibration procedure

The calibration of the system aims to achieve specific characteristics of the voluntary muscle signal, as each person may have a different muscle activity. Thus, the calibration allows that the system is generic and therefore adapts itself to different users. The calibration procedure of the system involves capturing the muscle signal in a time of relaxation and in a moment of maximum voluntary contraction (MVC).

Figure 11 shows a brief block diagram of the calibration procedure. This step involves eight Boolean variables (SNR (x), x = 1.2 .. 8) indicating that all channels of myoelectric signal acquisition were correctly calibrated. If a pair of electrodes is not properly positioned, the distress signal has low quality, and once again must be repositioned until the signal / noise ratio is at least greater than 2 - value established based on the signal acquisition trials previously conducted with this electromyograph (Favieiro, 2009).

For the calibration of each channel, initially an acquisition of the signal is performed with the muscle in rest position. Then the signal is processed to calculate the average peak values. Later on a MVC movement is performed and captured, and after this, again the average peak value is calculated. With this information is possible to evaluate the signal to noise ratio (SNR) that is given by dividing the value processed during the movement with MVC by the value found when captured a rest movement.

A percentage ranging from 30-50% of the average peak values of the acquired signal with the maximum voluntary contraction (MVC) is then used to determine, during processing of the signal, the threshold value which indicates whether or not a muscle contraction occurring during the process of windowing the signal.

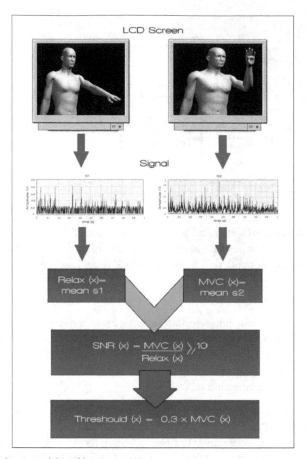

**Figure 11.** Block diagram of the calibration routine.

The movements with MVC used for the calibration of each channel are shown in the table 1.

| Channel x | Muscle | Movement |
|-----------|--------|----------|
| 0 | Biceps | Forearm flexion |
| 1 | Flexor carpi ulnaris | Hand abduction |
| 2 | Flexor carpi radialis | Hand adduction |
| 3 | Extensor digitorum | Hand contraction |
| 4 | Pronator teres | Forearm rotation |
| 5 | Brachioradialis | Forearm rotation |
| 6 | Palmaris longus | Wrist flexion |
| 7 | Extensor carpi ulnaris | Wrist extension |

**Table 1.** Representation of movement defined for each channel calibration.

## 3.4.2. Preprocessing procedures

Were used mathematical procedures typically used in the myoelectric signal analysis to preprocess the signal and generating one or more characteristics of interest to the classification stage.

The techniques used are this stage was (for further details consult Favieiro, 2011):

- removal of DC component (offset adjustment);
- full-wave rectification;
- windowing the signal of interest;
- determining the rms value of the signal of interest.

The signal is analyzed in periods of 50 ms, since it provides a comprehensive overview of the signal but, at the same time, specific, since it does not occur in tests muscle relaxation in period shorter than the determined, resulting in an efficient analysis of runtime system and results. To perform the windowing of the signal, the period in which a muscle contraction occurs were developed a routine in Labview which analyses the signal every 50 ms, where each channel is analyzed simultaneously, ensuring if in these data windows occurs a signal peak with value above the threshold. To consider that a movement is taking place is necessary to satisfy the following assumptions:

- is considered that the channel is active if, in the processed time window, there are any peaks above the threshold limit. Considering the threshold a variable that has a value ranging from 30-50% of the respective channel MVC. This percentage is defined empirically according to preliminary test conducted with a user;
- is necessary that at least three channels have a peak above the respective threshold, i.e., being active. This is done to ensure that any random noise introduced in at least one channel interfere with the signal windowing;
- the signal must be considered active, at least 80% of the last 20 windows, i.e., the last one second. The history of activation of the channels is taken into consideration to try to ensure that a movement is actually occurring.

With these assumptions satisfied, it is considered that a movement is occurring, and in turn, the signal is windowed in all channels simultaneously, considering the same time based for the beginning and end of the muscle contraction. Another assumption considered important is if two sequential movements were spaced in time by up to 3 seconds, they will be considered one single movement and the beginning time of the first movements and the end time of the second are used to define a new single window containing these two movements. Thus, ensuring that complex movements are not considered two or more distinct movements by the signal windowing.

The set time of 3 seconds has been based on in the resting time of the Subject, which is 3 seconds. Thus, the windowing of a movement is determined only after a time longer than 3 seconds without the occurrence of a movement, only then is possible to analyze the windows stored in each channel, calculating the rms value from each channel in the occurrence time of a muscle contraction.

## 3.5. Myoelectric signal preprocessing by the neuro fuzzy method

The step of characterizing the signal is achieved by a neuro fuzzy type ANFIS. The system takes as input the rms values of each pre-processed data acquisition channel. Presents as output the movements characterized that are being carried out by the human arm. The system ANFIS used in this research was implemented using the Matlab tool (Fuzzy Logic Toolbox). The fuzzy neural network is interfaced via Labview, where the routine developed in Matlab is called when needed, being processed in the background.

### 3.5.1. Neuro fuzzy network dimensioning

First was set the number of network inputs, which can vary from 2 to 8 depending on the number of channels which is intended to analyze. The channel that will be used on the network can be selected by the operator of the system which the developed routine performs reading of all channels and automatically separates the desired channels for processing. This function has as input the array of channels to be selected and as output only the desired channels. The output of the neuro-fuzzy networks is considered fixed, containing the 12 movements previously determined. The output values ranges from 0 to 1, and for each movement there is a corresponding fixed known value, as shown in Table 2.

He developed structure is a fuzzy network type Sugeno obtained in the generation of a initial structure adapted from a input-output set acquired in the systems tests. The structure contains eight inputs and one output.

| Movement | Corresponded output |
|---|---|
| Hand contraction | 0 |
| Wrist extension | 0.083 |
| Wrist flexion | 0.166 |
| Forearm flexion | 0.249 |
| Forearm rotation | 0.333 |
| Hand abduction | 0.416 |
| Hand adduction | 0.499 |
| Complex 1 | 0.582 |
| Complex 2 | 0.665 |
| Complex 3 | 0.748 |
| Complex 4 | 0.831 |
| Complex 5 | 0.914 |

**Table 2.** Network output values associated with the recognized movements.

### 3.5.2. Fuzzy neural network structure definition

To adjust the system it is necessary first creates an initial fuzzy network, which should be representative of the Subject data. For this, was used the subtractive clustering technique, which can generate, from a input-output data, membership functions of input and output, and the fuzzy rules structure for type Sugeno. This technique was chosen because it obtained good results in preliminary studies cases, its routine is represented in Figure 12. This routine is performed using the MatlabScript node that defines a script to be run in Matlab.

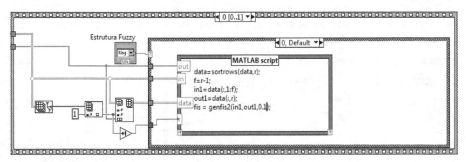

**Figure 12.** Routine developed for definition of the fuzzy network structure.

While creating the initial fuzzy structure was necessary to define the following parameters in Matlab:

- input data: array with fuzzy inputs of the network;
- output data: array with the expected output for the input data set;
- membership function: the Gaussian function was selected because it is a smooth function on the edges, have shown better results in these trials;
- radius: was selected the value of 0.1, which represents the influence radius of the cluster, when it is considered a unitary hypercube. The smaller the radius, more clusters are created and, consequentially, a greater number of rules.

In the first Subject assay, the expected input and output values are used to create the system initial structure representing the fuzzy network of 8 inputs, 60 clusters (i.e., 60 rules) e one output, generated for a system assay, and adjust it later to adapt to represent more faithfully a model that can characterize the Subject movements.

After creating the initial fuzzy structure is necessary to adapt the membership functions for the data acquired in the session, thus making a fine adjustment of the functions, leading to results more consistent with the ones expected. The adaptation step is very important, because it help to better define the limits and parameters of the membership functions, leaving the model best suited for the Subject. In this step were used a hybrid training function. The hybrid training is a combination of the gradient method with the LSE method to optimize the time convergence of the model, since it reduces the demand on the dimensional space. This function used the following parameters, according to the routine which utilized the MatlabScript function represented in Figure 13:

- initial fuzzy network, created from the subtractive clustering technique;
- input data: array with the network fuzzy inputs;
- output data: vector with the expected output for the input data set;

- number of training epochs: the value 10 was selected , which defines the number of training cycles, i.e., the maximum number of times the training set is presented to the network. An excessive number of cycles can lead to loss of power to the network generalization (over fitting). On the other hand, with a small number of cycles, the network cannot reach its best performance (under fitting);
- target error: the value 0 was selected, which consists in terminate the training after the mean square error falls below a predetermined value $\alpha$.

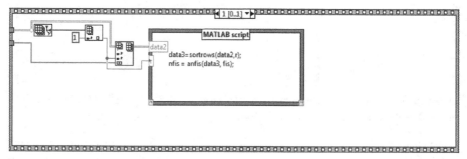

**Figure 13.** Training routine of the neuro-fuzzy network.

As output of the training step, is generated a fuzzy network with adapted membership functions to a particular Subject, causing the limits of each functions to be left according to the training data.

## 4. Results and discussion

This topic will discuss the test performed during system development, and the results obtained. It is important to note that the pre-processing routine and calibration have already been validated in previous studies (Favieiro, 2009; Favieiro & Balbinot, 2011).

Subjects participating in this research present an age range of 20±5 years old, of both sexes. Altogether were conducted trials with seven Subjects. The abbreviations of the characterized movements are presented in Table 3.

It is worth noting that the parameters of ANFIS training were the same for all Subjects. Figure 14 represents the result of section 2 for Subject 1 where is possible notice that for the movement M11 that is the hand contraction with the forearm flexion, 40% of the error was due to the fact that the network believed was dealing with movement M0 (hand contraction) which represents partially the movement performed. Another movement in which occurred the incorrect recognition was the M4 (forearm rotation) with M3 (forearm flexion), causing 60% of error, which may occur since these movements uses muscle in common, such as the biceps, and were used only surface electrodes.

As an example, Table 4 represents the average accuracy rate of the system for each movement per session, and the overall average of each movement per session for the Subject 1. The movements with lower hit rate are: hand contraction (M0), forearm rotation (M4) and hand contraction and forearm rotation (M11), with 65%, 57% and 50% hit rate, respectively. It happened by the similarity of M4 to M3 (forearm flexion) and by the similarity between M0 to M11.

| Performed movement | Abbreviation |
|---|---|
| Hand contraction | M0 |
| Wrist extension | M1 |
| Wrist flexion | M2 |
| Forearm flexion | M3 |
| Forearm rotation | M4 |
| Hand abduction | M5 |
| Hand adduction | M6 |
| Hand contraction with forearm rotation | M7 |
| Forearm rotation and flexion | M8 |
| Forearm rotation and flexion with wrist flexion | M9 |
| Wrist extension followed by flexion | M10 |
| Hand contraction with forearm flexion | M11 |

**Table 3.** Abbreviations representing the performed movements.

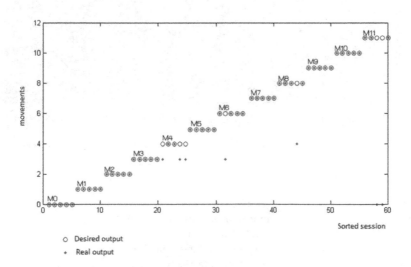

**Figure 14.** System output for Subject 1 – section 2 (5 repetitions).

| Subject 1 | M0 | M1 | M2 | M3 | M4 | M5 | M6 | M7 | M8 | M9 | M10 | M11 |
|---|---|---|---|---|---|---|---|---|---|---|---|---|
| Session 2 (%) | 100 | 100 | 100 | 100 | 40 | 100 | 80 | 100 | 80 | 100 | 100 | 60 |
| Session 3 (%) | 40 | 100 | 80 | 80 | 60 | 60 | 100 | 80 | 100 | 100 | 80 | 80 |
| Session 4 (%) | 60 | 80 | 100 | 80 | 80 | 80 | 100 | 100 | 80 | 100 | 40 | 20 |
| Session 5 (%) | 60 | 100 | 100 | 100 | 50 | 100 | 20 | 100 | 40 | 60 | 60 | 40 |
| Average (%) | 65 | 95 | 95 | 90 | 57 | 85 | 75 | 95 | 75 | 90 | 70 | 50 |

**Table 4.** Summary of the system average accuracy rate to the subject 1.

## 4.1. Comparison between subjects

As an example, Figure 15 shows the average accuracy rate for movement M10 for all Subjects. The average score was higher than 70% in all cases. This happened mainly because of the simple movements that compose the M10 movement are easily detectable antagonistic movements. Like the movements M1 and M2 achieved accuracy rates above 75% in most cases.

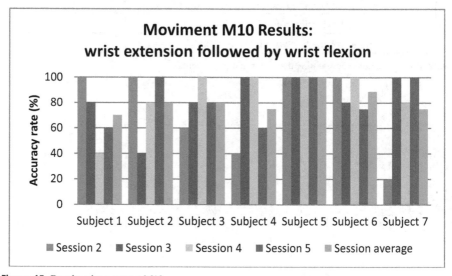

**Figure 15.** Results of movement M10.

Figure 16 represents the average of all tests performed for each movement. Analyzing the graph it is clear that the more accurate movements were M1, M2, M5 and M10 (combination of M1 and M2), with averages rates of approximately 80%. These movements are quite distinct, which increases the accuracy rate of the system. The worst case occurred with the movement M11, which had an average hit rate below 50%, it combines simple movements used in most of the complex movements performed, impairing the correct recognition. Overall the system achieved an average accuracy of 65%.

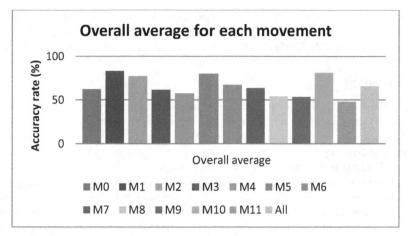

**Figure 16.** Overall result of the system for each movement.

## 4.2. Comparison between the researched results and other studies

The vast majority of studies in the area of recognition of hand-movements of the arm segment are based on the classification of simple movements, not taking into account combined movements, as was the aim of this study. As it was possible to see the results of this work, most of the errors were caused by similar movements, or the differentiation of compound movements with their simple movements. The human arm has many degrees of freedom and be able to develop a system that can characterize many different movements and combined is where the real challenge and for this reason is an active area of research (Favieiro et al., 2011; Favieiro & Balbinot, 2011).

Comparing the system developed by Chan using fuzzy techniques which were classified four simple movements using only two channels with an accuracy of 91% (Chan, 2000). Also a system was developed by Ajiboye to characterize four classes of movements using four channels, obtaining an accuracy of 86% (Ajiboye, 2005). These systems had similar results to those found in the preliminary study of this research in which the neuro fuzzy technique was used to classify five distinct movements using three channels of signal acquisition, obtaining an accuracy of 86% (Favieiro & Balbinot, 2011). Demonstrating the system using only simple movements and a limited number of channels achieved accuracy higher than that found to characterize the combined movements.

Compared with the research of Momen which categorize nine distinct movements, using only the rms characteristic of the window processed and four acquisition channels obtained an average accuracy of 48.9%. This study is very similar to the system developed, in the sense that uses the same characteristic of the signal and making a direct comparison of the average hit rate of the developed system is 30% higher than to 9 moves obtained per Momen (Momen, 2007).

Another difference that it is important to note is that the proposed study used only one feature extracted for each channel, unlike other studies that use up to 13 features per channel, whose average accuracy was 87% for the classification of 10 distinct movements (Khushaba, 2010).

## 5. Conclusions

The proposed system was designed to use a limited amount of up to 8 channels of the myoelectric signal acquisition and with the assistance of a more robust artificial intelligence technique was able to verify the validity of this system in terms of performance in the characterization of 11 distinct movements, including 5 complex movements. In tests, the mean peak signal with a maximum voluntary contraction (MVC) appeared at least four times greater than the average peak signal at a time of muscle relaxation. Thus, was possible determine a level ranging from 30 to 50% of MVC to differentiate a time of muscle contraction, representing a movement. With the windowing signal occurs at the instant when a movement occurs, is possible to obtain the rms value for each of the channels 8 and to use these values as input to a neuro fuzzy network with one output an up to 8 inputs. This network aims to characterize the movements that are being executed. The network is adapted in accordance with supervised training, to evaluate system performance over time. As can be seen on the results, some movements have achieved a lower hit rate, this may occur due to poor signal quality, user error, and the quantity of motion that was presented to the neuro fuzzy network, since most of the errors were caused by similar movements, or the differentiation of compound movements with their simple movements, which have a response very similar in rms value, causing the network to get confused. The average accuracy obtained was 65% of hit rate to 11 distinct movements in tests of long duration, about three hours.

Also, it's important to notice that the vast majority of studies in the area of recognition of hand-movements of the arm segment are based on the classification of simple movements, not taking into account combined movements, as was the aim of this study. The preliminary study of this research in which the neuro fuzzy technique was used to classify five distinct simple movements using three channels of signal acquisition, obtained an accuracy of 86% (Favieiro & Balbinot, 2011). Demonstrating the system using only simple movements and a limited number of channels achieved accuracy higher than that found to characterize the combined movements.

The human arm has many degrees of freedom and be able to develop a system that can characterize many different movements and combined is the real challenge of this kind of research, which will really improve the life quality of people with special needs, making them more independent and more likely to real social and economical integration.

## 6. Future studies

It would be very important in future studies performing the tests with a larger number of volunteers, to conduct a robust statistical analysis of results, and allow a more robust assessment of its results, its flaws and strengths. Is ongoing the use of the system with Volunteers with total and partial amputation of the upper limb. This is crucial for research to find out how the system would apply and adapt, it is possible to ascertain the validity of future control system for a prosthetic hand-arm segment by myoelectric signals. Another proposal for further work would find other characteristics that could be extracted from the signal to improve the performance of the fuzzy neural network, so that the system would be able to characterize a wide range of complex movements with a hit ratio above 90%, and a higher capacity to differentiate motion. One way to improve the hit rate of the system is to implement a feedback to the user, to the person performing the test whether they are doing it correctly, avoiding common errors of distraction, or applying excessive force.

## Author details

Gabriela Winkler Favieiro and Alexandre Balbinot
*Federal University of Rio Grande do Sul (UFRGS)*
*Graduate Program in Electrical Engineering (PPGEE), Department of Electrical Engineering,*
*Instrumentation Laboratory, Porto Alegre, Rio Grande do Sul, Brazil*

## 7. References

Ajiboye, A.B. & Weir, R.F. (2005). A heuristic fuzzy logic approach to EMG pattern recognition for multifunctional prosthesis control. *IEEE Transactions on Neural Systems and Rehabilitation Engineering*, Baltimore, V.13, No.3, pp. 280–291.

Balbinot, A. (2006). Desenvolvimento de uma Prótese experimental controlada por eletromiografia. *Proceedings of Congresso Ibero-Americano sobre Tecnologias de Apoio a Portadores de Dediciência*, Vitória, IBERDISCAP, 2006, V.1, MA-3–MA-6.

Begg R.K., Lai D. & Palaniswami M (2008). Computational Intelligence in Biomedical Engineering, Taylor & Francis Books Inc (CRC Press), Boca Raton, Florida, USA (392 pages), ISBN: 0-8493-4080-2.

Chan, F.H.Y (2000). Fuzzy EMG classification for prosthesis control. *IEEE Transactions on Neural Systems and Rehabilitation Engineering*, Baltimore, V.8, No. 3, pp. 305–311.

Chiu, S. L. (1994). Fuzzy model identification based on cluster estimation. *Journal of Intelligent and Fuzzy systems*, V.2, No. 3, pp. 267-278.

DeConto, E. & Balbinot, A. (2011). Desenvolvimento de modelos virtuais para EMG. Relatório de Pesquisa, Porto Alegre, UFRGS.

Dubois, D. & Prade, H. (1980). *Fuzzy set and systems: theory and applications*. New York: Academic Press.

Englehart, K. & Hudgins, B. (2003). A robust, real-time control scheme for multifunction myoelectric control. *IEEE Transactions on Biomedical Engineering*, Gainesville, V. 50, No. 7, pp. 848–854.

Favieiro, G. & Balbinot, A. (2011). Adaptive Neuro-Fuzzy Logic Analysis Based on Myoelectric Signals for Multifunction Prosthesis Control, *Proceedings of Annual International Conference of the IEEE Engineering in Medicine and Biology Society 2011*, pp. 7888-7891, Boston, EMBS, 2011.

Favieiro, G. (2009). *Controle de uma prótese experimental do segmento mão-braço por sinais mioelétricos e redes neurais artificiais*. 2009. 111 f. Trabalho de conclusão de curso. Engenharia de computação, Universidade Federal do Rio Grande do Sul, Porto Alegre.

Favieiro, G.; Balbinot, A. & Barreto, M.M.G. (2011). Decoding arm movements by myoeletric signals and artificial neural networks. *Proceedings of Biosignals and Biorobotics Conferecene (BRC) 2011*, pp. 1-6, Vitória, ISSNIP, 2011.

Hincapie, J.G. & Kirsch, R.F. (2009). Feasibility of EMG-Based neural network controller for an upper extremity neuroprosthesis. *IEEE Transactions on Biomedical Engineering*, Gainesville, V.17, No. 1, pp. 80–90.

Hudgins, B.; Parker, p. & Scott, R. (1994). Control of artificial limbs using myoelectric pattern recognition. *Medical and Life Sciences Engineering*, pp. 21-38.

Hudgins, B.; Parker, P. & Scott, R.N. (1991). A neural network classifier for multifunction myoelectric control. *Proceedings of International Confercence IEEE-EMBS*, Orlando, EMBS, 1991, V.13, No..3, pp. 1454-1455.

Jacobsen, S; Knutti, D.; Johnson R & Sears, H. (1982). Development of the Utah artificial arm. *IEEE Transactions on Biomedical Engineering*, No. 29, pp. 249-269.

Jang, J.R. (1993). ANFIS: adaptive-network-based fuzzy inference systems. *IEEE Transactions on systems, Man, and Cybernetics*, V. 23, No. 3, pp. 665-685.

Jang, J.R.; Sun, C. & Mizutani, E. (1997). *Neuro-fuzzy and soft computing: a computational approach to learning and machine intelligence*. New York: Prentice Hall.

Katutoshi, K.; Koji, O. & Takao, T. (1992). A discrimination system using neural network for EMG-controlled prosthesies. *Proceedings of the IEEE International Workshop on Robot Human Communication*, No. 1, pp. 63-68.

Khushaba, R.N.; Al-Ani, A. & Al-Jumaily, A. (2010). Orthogonal Fuzzy Neighborhood discriminant analysis for multifunction myoeletric hand control. *IEEE Transactions on Biomedical Engineering*, Gainesville, V.57, No. .6, pp. 1410–1419.

Li, G.; Schultz, A.E. & Kuizen, T. A. (2010). Quantifying pattern recognition: based myoeletric control of multifunctional transradial prosthesis. *IEEE Transactions on Neural Systems and Rehabilitation Engineering*, V. 18, No.. 2, pp. 185–192.

Momen, K.; Krishnan, S. & Chau, T. (2007). Real-time classification of forearm electromyographic signals corresponding to user-selected intentional movements for multifunction prosthesis control. *IEEE Transactions on Neural Systems and Rehabilitation Engineering*, Baltimore, V.15, No. .4, pp. 535–542.

Park, E. & Meek, S. (1995). Adaptive filtering of the electromyographic signal for prosthetic control and force estimation. *IEEE Transactions on Biomedical Engineering*, Vol. 42, No. 10, pp. 1048-1052.

Rutkowski, L & Cpalka, K. (2005). Designing and learning of adjustable quasi-triangular norms with applications to neuro-fuzzy systems. *IEEE Trans. on Fuzzy Systems*, V. 14, No. 1, pp. 140-151.

Sugeno, M. & Kang, G. T. (1988). Structure identification of fuzzy model. *Fuzzy Sets and Systems*, North Holland, V.28, N.3, pp. 15-33.

Takagi, T. & Sugeno, M. (1985). Fuzzy identification of systems and its applications to modeling and control. *IEEE Transactions on Systems, Man, and Cybertnetics*, New York, V.15, No. 1, pp. 116-132.

Zadeh, L., M. Nikravesh, & Loia V. (2004). *Fuzzy logic and the Internet. Studies in fuzziness and soft computing*, Vol. 137. Berlin, Springer.

# Chapter 10

# Signal Acquisition Using Surface EMG and Circuit Design Considerations for Robotic Prosthesis

Muhammad Zahak Jamal

Additional information is available at the end of the chapter

## 1. Introduction

Electromyography (EMG) is the subject which deals with the detection, analysis and utilization of electrical signals emanating from skeletal muscles. The field of electromyography is studied in Biomedical Engineering. And prosthesis using electromyography is achieved under Biomechatronics [1]. The electric signal produced during muscle activation, known as the myoelectric signal, is produced from small electrical currents generated by the exchange of ions across the muscle membranes and detected with the help of electrodes. Electromyography is used to evaluate and record the electrical activity produced by muscles of a human body. The instrument from which we obtain the EMG signal is known as electromyograph and the resultant record obtained is known as electromyogram [2].

The human body is a wonder of nature. The functioning of human body is an intriguing and fascinating activity. Motion of the human body is a perfect integration of the brain, nervous system and muscles. It is altogether a well-organized effort of the brain with 28 major muscles to control the trunk and limb joints to produce forces needed to counter gravity and propel the body forward with minimum amount of energy expenditure [3]. The movement of the human body is possible through muscles in coordination with the brain. Whenever the muscles of the body are to be recruited for a certain activity, the brain sends excitation signals through the Central Nervous System (CNS). Muscles are innervated in groups called 'Motor Units'. A motor unit is the junction point where the motor neuron and the muscle fibers meet. A depiction of the Motor Unit is given in Figure 1. When the motor unit is activated, it produces a 'Motor Unit Action Potential' (MUAP) [4]. The activation from the Central Nervous System is repeated continuously for as long as the muscle is required to generate force. This continued activation produces motor unit action potential trains. The trains from concurrently active motor units superimpose to produce the resultant EMG signal. A group of muscles are involved in a certain movement of the human body. The number of muscles recruited depends upon the activity in which the body is involved. E.g. in lifting a small weight such as a tiny pebble, fewer amount of muscles will be involved as compared to lifting a heavy mass like a 6 kg weight, where the muscles employed will be greater. In technical terms, whenever it is required to generate greater force, the excitation from the Central Nervous System increases, more motor units are activated and the firing rate of all the motor units increase resulting in high EMG signal amplitudes [4,5].

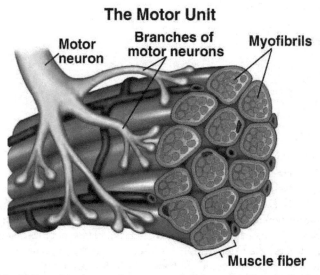

**Figure 1.** A Motor Unit consists of one motor neuron and all the muscle fibers it stimulates [6]

Electromyography enables us to generate force, create movements and allow us to do countless other functions through which we can interact with the world around us. The electromyograph is a bioelectric signal which has, over the years, developed a vast range of applications. Clinically, electromyography is being used as diagnostic tool for neurological disorders. It is frequently being used for assessment of patients with neuromuscular diseases, low back pain and disorders of motor control [7]. Other than physiological and biomechanical research, EMG has been developed as an evaluation tool in applied research, physiotherapy, rehabilitation, sports medicine and training, biofeedback and ergonomics research.

In the recent past, EMG has also found its use in rehabilitation of patients with amputations in the form of robotic prosthesis. EMG proves to be a valuable tool as it provides a natural way of sensing and classifying different movements of the body. A multi-degree of freedom robotic mechanism can effectively imitate the motion of the human limb. Recent advances in electronics and microcontroller technology have allowed improved control options for robotic mechanisms. One of the most vital advantages of microprocessor technology in robotic prosthetics is the advanced EMG filtering algorithms. Nowadays, control options are even available to those who were not at one time qualified for such prosthetic management.

This chapter will discuss in detail, the effective use of surface electromyography (SEMG) as a tool for achieving robotic prosthesis. An elaborate account of SEMG electrode types, signal acquisition technique, electronics circuit design considerations and the control procedure to drive electric motors in a robotic mechanism is provided in this chapter.

## 2. EMG electrodes and its types

The bioelectrical activity inside the muscle of a human body is detected with the help of EMG electrodes. There are two main types of EMG electrodes: surface (or skin electrodes) and inserted electrodes. Inserted electrodes have further two types: needle and fine wire electrodes. The three electrodes (needle, fine wire and surface) are explained as follows. Among these three electrodes, surface EMG electrodes will be specifically discussed in detail as it pertains to the topic of this chapter.

### 2.1. Needle electrodes

Needle electrodes are widely used in clinical procedures in neuromuscular evaluations. The tip of the needle electrode is bare and used as a detection surface. It contains an insulated wire in the cannula. The signal quality from the needle electrodes is comparatively improved from other available types. Needle electrodes have two main advantages. One is that its relatively small pickup area enables the electrode to detect individual MUAPs during relatively low force contractions. The other is that the electrodes may be conveniently repositioned within the muscle (after insertion) so that new tissue territories may be explored [5]. A needle electrode is shown in Figure 2.

### Concentric Needle Electrodes

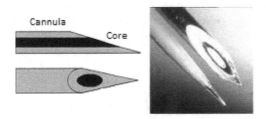

**Figure 2.** A Needle EMG Electrode [8]

### 2.2. Fine wire electrodes

Wire electrodes are made from any small diameter, highly non-oxidizing, stiff wire with insulation. Alloys of platinum, silver, nickel, and chromium are typically used. Wire electrodes are extremely fine, they are easily implanted and withdrawn from skeletal muscles, and they are generally less painful than needle electrodes whose cannula remains inserted in the muscle throughout the duration of the test [5]. A fine wire electrode is shown in Figure 3.

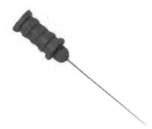

**Figure 3.** Fine Wire EMG Electrode

## 2.3. Surface EMG electrode

Surface EMG electrodes provide a non-invasive technique for measurement and detection of EMG signal. The theory behind these electrodes is that they form a chemical equilibrium between the detecting surface and the skin of the body through electrolytic conduction, so that current can flow into the electrode.

These electrodes are simple and very easy to implement. Application of needle and fine wire electrodes require strict medical supervision and certification. Surface EMG electrodes require no such formalities. Surface EMG electrodes have found their use in motor behavior studies, neuromuscular recordings, sports medical evaluations [9] and for subjects who object to needle insertions such as children. Apart from all this, surface EMG is being increasingly used to detect muscle activity in order to control device extensions to achieve prosthesis for physically disabled and amputated population.

Surface EMG has some limitations as well. Since these electrodes are applied on the skin, hence, they are generally used for superficial muscles only. Crosstalk from other muscles is a major problem. Their position must be kept stable with the skin; otherwise, the signal is distorted.

### 2.3.1. Types of EMG Electrodes

There are two types of surface EMG electrodes: Gelled and Dry EMG electrodes [10].

#### 2.3.1.1. Gelled EMG Electrodes

Gelled EMG electrodes contain a gelled electrolytic substance as an interface between skin and electrodes. Oxidation and reduction reactions take place at the metal electrode junction. Silver – silver chloride (Ag-AgCl) is the most common composite for the metallic part of gelled electrodes. The AgCl layer allows current from the muscle to pass more freely across the junction between the electrolyte and the electrode. This introduces less electrical noise into the measurement, as compared with equivalent metallic electrodes (e.g. Ag). Due to this fact, Ag-AgCl electrodes are used in over 80% of surface EMG applications [10].

Disposable gelled EMG electrodes are most common; however, reusable gelled electrodes are also available. Special skin preparations and precautions such as (hair removal, proper gel concentration, prevention of sweat accumulation etc.) are required for gelled electrodes in order to acquire the best possible signal. Gelled EMG electrodes are shown in Figure 4.

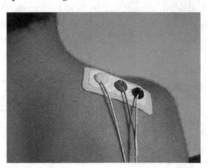

**Figure 4.** Gelled EMG Electrodes

*2.3.1.2. Dry EMG electrodes*

Dry EMG electrodes do not require a gel interface between skin and the detecting surface. Bar electrodes and array electrodes are examples of dry electrodes. These electrodes may contain more than one detecting surface. In many examples, an in-house pre-amplification circuitry may also be employed in these electrodes. A reusable bar electrode is shown in Figure 5. Dry electrodes are usually heavier (>20g) as compared to gelled electrodes (<1g). This increased inertial mass can cause problems for electrode fixation; therefore, a material for stability of the electrode with the skin is required [10].

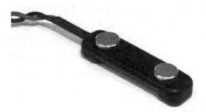

**Figure 5.** A Reusable Bar Electrode (an Example of Dry EMG Electrode)

### 2.3.2.Categories of Surface EMG Electrodes

There are two categories of surface EMG electrodes [5]: Passive and Active EMG electrodes. They are briefly explained as follows:-

*2.3.2.1. Passive EMG electrodes*

These electrodes should be connected to an external amplification circuitry with the help of connecting wires for the proper acquisition of the EMG signal. Passive EMG electrodes can be disposable or reusable.

Electrodes shown in Figure 4 and Figure 5 both fall under passive surface EMG electrodes.

*2.3.2.2. Active EMG electrodes*

Active EMG electrodes contain a pre-amplifier attachment for surface electrodes. Needle and fine wire surface electrodes are also available. These electrodes usually fall under the dry surface EMG electrodes type. The in-house high impedance amplifier in these electrodes transfers the pre-amplified signal to the rest of the circuitry. Figure 6 shows an active EMG electrode.

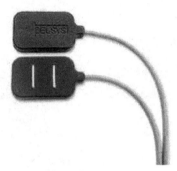

**Figure 6.** The Delsys 2.1 Active EMG Electrode [11]

## 3. EMG electrode placement and signal acquisition technique

Surface EMG is relatively easy to use as compared to other EMG electrodes. This is the reason why it is being extensively used in the control of robotic mechanisms to achieve prosthesis. It is also widely used in latest EMG researches by engineers as no medical certification or expertise is required for its application. Its use in rehabilitation prosthesis is favorable as it does not cause any kind of discomfort to the subject on whom it is applied. Other kinds of EMG electrodes (needle and fine wire), when inserted into the skin of the subject, may effect a twitching sensation and cause him or her to make movements.

In order to get the best results from SEMG, it is really important to have a proper understanding of the muscles from which the EMG signal is being extracted. The placement on skin also requires adequate study and requires skin preparation beforehand as well.

The EMG electrodes, their types, sub-types and categories have already been explained in detail in the previous section. Since, our concern is only with Surface EMG (SEMG), hence, we will only deal with the placement and signal acquisition technique using surface EMG electrodes.

### 3.1. Overview of muscle architecture

Skeletal muscle architecture is defined in terms of "the arrangement of muscle fibers relative to the axis of force generation." The skeletal muscle arrangement as well as their activity reveals striking organization at the macroscopic level. The functional properties of the skeletal muscle depend strongly on their architecture [12].

There are various kinds of muscle fiber arrangements, which are discussed as follows:-

i.   Muscles with fibers that extend parallel to the muscle force-generating axis are termed **parallel, fusiform** or **longitudinally** arranged muscles. Examples of such types of muscles are Biceps Brachii (bicep muscle) and Sartorius (groin muscle).

ii.  Muscles with fibers that are oriented at a single angle relative to the force generating axis are termed **unipennate** muscles. Example of unipennate muscle is Extensor Digitorum Longus.

iii. The angle between the fiber and the force-generating axis generally varies from 0° to 30°. The muscles are oriented at more than one angle. Most muscles fall into this category and they are called as **multipennate** muscles. Examples are Rectus Femoris which is bipennate and Deltoid which is multipennate.

iv.  The muscles which surround an opening so as to form a closed shape are known as **circular** muscles. Example of such kind of muscle is Orbicularis Oris (mouth muscle).

v.   The muscles in which their fibers converge on the insertion to maximize force of contraction are known as **Convergent** muscles. E.g. Pectoralis Major.

A detailed depiction of these muscle arrangements is provided in Figure 7.

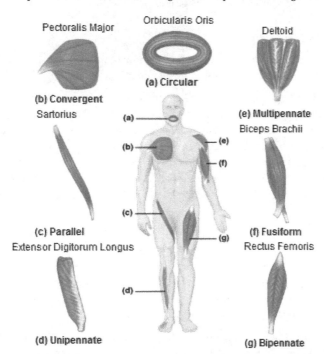

**Figure 7.** Muscles and their Architecture [13]

## 3.2. Skin preparation

Application of surface EMG electrodes requires proper skin preparation beforehand. In order to obtain a good quality EMG signal, the skin's impedance must be considerably reduced. For this purpose, the dead cells on the skin e.g. hair must be completely removed from the location where the EMG electrodes are to be placed. It is advisable to use an abrasive gel to reduce the dry layer of the skin [9]. There should be no moisture on the skin. The skin should be cleaned with alcohol in order to eliminate any wetness or sweat on the skin.

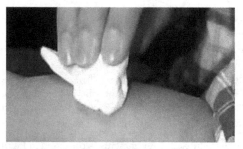

**Figure 8.** Skin Preparation prior to application of EMG electrodes

## 3.3. EMG electrode placement

The application of EMG electrodes requires adequate know how of the skeletal muscles. The EMG electrode placement will be discussed in detail under this section.

In most cases, two detecting surfaces (or EMG electrodes) are placed on the skin in bipolar configuration [14, 15]. In order to acquire the best possible signal, the EMG electrode should be placed at a proper location and its orientation across the muscle is important. The surface EMG electrodes should be placed between the motor unit and the tendinous insertion of the muscle, along the longitudinal midline of the muscle [15]. The distance between the center of the electrodes or detecting surfaces should only be 1-2 cm. The longitudinal axis of the electrodes (which passes through both detecting surfaces) should be parallel to the length of the muscle fibers.

As mentioned previously, the EMG detecting surfaces should be placed in between the motor unit and the tendon insertion of the muscle. Detecting surfaces placed on the belly of the muscle has proved to be a more than acceptable location. Here, the target muscle fiber density is the highest [15]. Figure 9 shows the proper EMG electrode placement. When the electrodes are arranged in this way, the detecting surfaces intersect most of the same muscle fibers, and as a result, an improved superimposed signal is observed.

The electrodes should not be placed elsewhere. In the past, a misconception prevailed that the EMG detecting surfaces should be placed on the motor unit. But, as a matter of fact, the electrode location on the motor point serves as the worst location for signal detection [15].

Similarly, the electrodes should neither be placed at or near the tendon nor at the edge of the muscle. The muscle fibers become thinner and smaller in number when they approach the tendon of the muscle resulting in a weak EMG signal, proving the fact that electrode placement near the tendon is not feasible. If the electrode is placed at the edge of the muscle, the chances of crosstalk from other muscles will considerably increase, and the resultant signal will be disturbed by those of other muscles [15].

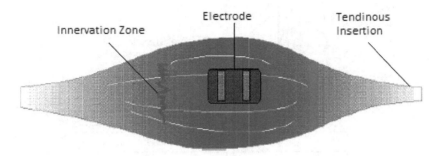

**Figure 9.** The ideal position of the electrode (two detecting surfaces) is between the innervation zone (or motor unit) and the tendinous insertion (or belly of the muscle) [15]

## 3.4. General concerns

Before we move on to the signal acquisition phase, it is very important to get acquainted with the EMG signal and the various concerns and factors affecting the qualitative properties of the signal.

The EMG signal's amplitude lies in between 1-10 mV, making it a considerably weak signal. The signal lies in the frequency range from 0-500 Hz and most dominant in between 50-150 Hz [15].

The EMG signal is highly influenced by noise [16], as shown in Figure 10. The characteristics of electrical noise can be caused from various sources. Ambient noise can be caused by electromagnetic radiation sources e.g. radio transmission devices, fluorescent lights and power line interference from electrical wires. These interferences are almost impossible to avoid from external means. This particular noise exists in the frequency range of 50-60 Hz. Noise can also be generated from motion artifact. The two main sources of this noise are instability of electrode skin interface and movement of the electrode cable and lies mostly in the range of 0-20 Hz. It can be eliminated by proper set of EMG equipment and circuitry. The maximum fidelity of the signal is determined by the acquired EMG signal-to-noise ratio [5, 14].

## 3.5. Reference electrode placement

The signal from the EMG detecting surfaces is gathered with respect to a reference. An EMG reference electrode acts as a ground for this signal. It should be placed far from the EMG detecting surfaces, on an electrically neutral tissue [15].

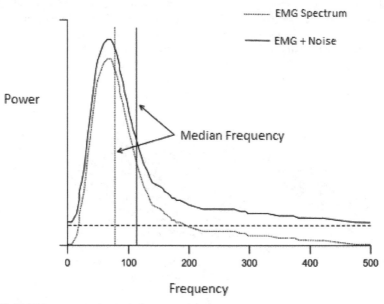

**Figure 10.** EMG Spectrum and noise influence on this spectrum [16]

## 3.6. EMG signal acquisition circuitry and configurations

The EMG electrode placement has been elaborately explained under the previous heading. So, after properly understanding the target muscle profile, preparing the skin and positioning the EMG detecting surfaces, comes the EMG signal acquisition step.

EMG signal is acquired through differential amplification technique. The differential amplifier should have high input impedance and very low output impedance. Ideally, a differential amplifier has infinite input and zero output impedance [17].

Differential amplification is achieved with the help of an instrumentation amplifier for high input impedance. A classic three amplifier instrumentation amplifier is shown in Figure 11.

The instrumentation amplifier carries out differential amplification by subtracting the voltages $V_1$ and $V_2$. This way, the noise signal which is common at $V_1$ and $V_2$ (electrode inputs) e.g. power line interference etc. are eliminated. The tendency of a differential amplification to reject signals common to both inputs is determined by common mode rejection ratio (CMRR). A CMRR of 90 dB is enough for elimination of common signals for instrumentation amplifiers, but latest technology, even though expensive, provides us with a CMRR of 120 dB. But there are reasons for not pushing the CMRR to the limit, as the electrical noise detected by the electrodes may not be in phase [15]. The gain for the instrumentation amplifier can be set using a single resistor ($R_{gain}$). The gain equation and output equation of the instrumentation amplifier is given in Eq. 1 and 2.

$$Gain = \left(1 + \frac{2R1}{Rgain}\right)\frac{R3}{R2} \tag{1}$$

$$Vout = (V2 - V1) \times Gain \tag{2}$$

A small gain of 5 or 6 is recommended for signal acquisition. Extensive amplification will be carried out in further steps. The placement of the EMG detecting surfaces can be done through three different configurations: monopolar, bipolar and multipolar.

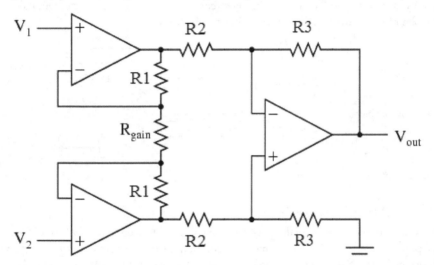

**Figure 11.** A Three Amplifier Instrumentation Amplifier

### 3.6.1. Monopolar configuration

The monopolar configuration is implemented using only a single electrode on the skin with respect to a reference electrode as shown in Figure 12. This method is used because of its simplicity, but is strictly not recommended as it detects all the electrical signals in the vicinity of the detecting surface [5, 14].

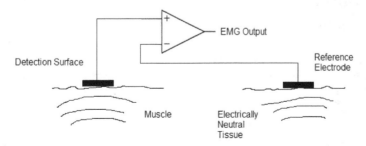

**Figure 12.** Monopolar signal acquisition technique

### 3.6.2. Bipolar configuration

Bipolar configuration is used to acquire EMG signal using two EMG detecting surfaces with the help of a reference electrode. The signals from the two EMG surfaces are connected to a differential amplifier. The two detecting surfaces are placed only 1-2 cm from each other. The differential amplifier suppresses the common noise signals to both inputs and then amplifies the difference [5, 14]. The limitations of the monopolar configuration are catered for by this configuration. This is the most commonly used electrode configuration. The bipolar EMG electrode configuration is shown is Figure 13.

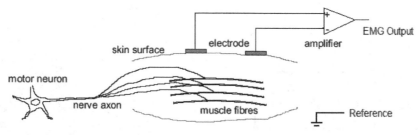

**Figure 13.** Bipolar Configuration

### 3.6.3. Multipolar configurations

This configuration uses more than two detecting surfaces to acquire the EMG signal with the help of a reference electrode. This configuration further reduces crosstalk and noise concerns [14]. A much more enhanced EMG signal is acquired from this configuration. The signals from three or more EMG detecting surfaces, placed 1-2 cm from each other, are passed through more than two stages of differential amplification. For example if three detecting surfaces are used then double differential technique is employed.

This configuration is   used in comprehensive researches carried out to study EMG muscle fiber orientation, conduction velocity and motor point localization.

## 4. Electrical design considerations

This section will discuss the electrical design considerations in order to synthesize the best possible EMG signal from the muscles of the human body in thorough detail. The basic circuitry for signal acquisition or preamplification circuitry is explained in due detail in the previous section. In this section we will discuss the circuitry implemented after the preamplification stage.

### 4.1. Filtering

As discussed earlier, there are many concerns regarding the proper detection of the EMG signal. Once the electrode is properly placed and the signal is extracted, noise plays a major role in hampering the recording of the EMG signal. For this purpose, the signal has to be properly filtered, even after differential amplification [18, 19].

The noise frequencies contaminating the raw EMG signal can be high as well as low. Low frequency noise can be caused from amplifier DC offsets, sensor drift on skin and temperature fluctuations and can be removed using a high pass filter. High frequency noise can be caused from nerve conduction and high frequency interference from radio broadcasts, computers, cellular phones etc. and can be deleted using a low pass filter.

In order to remove these high and low frequencies, high pass and low pass bio-filters will be discussed in adequate detail in this section.

### 4.1.1. High pass filter

A high pass filter is used to remove low frequency component from a particular electrical signal. A term 'cut-off frequency', denoted by '$f_c$', is the frequency below which all frequencies are eliminated. All frequencies above $f_c$ are carried forward. The frequency range where the filter response is '1' and the signals are transmitted is known as 'passband' region. On the contrary, the frequency range where the filter response is '0' and the signals are attenuated is known as 'stop band' region [18]. A high pass filter response is shown in Figure 14.

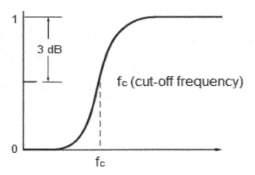

**Figure 14.** A high pass filter response

A high pass filter can be developed by using a resistor and a capacitor. This circuit will then be known as a CR circuit [20]. This circuit is a first order high pass filter. It is the simplest high pass filter possible. The high pass filtered signal is gathered across the resistor. The filter is shown in Figure 15.

The cut-off frequency of the high pass filter is given in Eq. 3.

$$fc = \frac{1}{2\pi RC} \tag{3}$$

A second order high pass filter can also be designed. An effective design can employ an active electronic component [20]. The design uses two first order filters in series and is facilitated by an operational amplifier. The circuit is given Figure 16.

For this circuit, if $R_1 = R_2$; $C_1 = C_2$ then $f_c$ is given as:-

$$fc = \frac{1}{2\pi RC} \tag{4}$$

$R_3$ and $R_4$ are optional and are required for separate gain settings as:-

$$A_0 = 1 + R_4/R_3 \tag{5}$$

Using a 2nd order filter is recommended as they provide a roll-off of 40 dB/dec as compared to 20 dB/dec provided by 1st order filters [18]. The use of active components can isolate the filter from the rest of the circuitry.

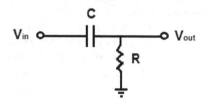

**Figure 15.** First order high pass filter

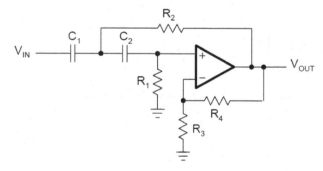

**Figure 16.** A 2nd Order High Pass Filter

## 4.1.2. Low pass filters

The concept of low pass filters is entirely opposite to that of high pass filters. In these filters, the frequencies less than the cut-off frequency are transmitted and above that are removed [18]. A low pass filter response is shown in Figure 17.

The simplest low pass filter can be designed with the help of a resistor and a capacitor called as a 1st order RC circuit [20]. The low pass filtered signal is detected across the capacitor. The 1st order low pass filter circuit is shown in Figure 18.

## Low Pass Filter

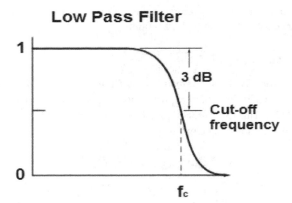

Figure 17. Low Pass Filter Response

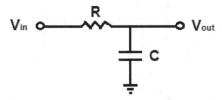

Figure 18. 1st Order Low Pass Filter

The cut-off frequency equation for the circuit in Figure 18 is the same as that of Eq. 3.

A 2nd order low pass filter can be more effective as compared to a 1st order one. It can be designed by cascading two 1st order filters attached to an operational amplifier. The circuit is given in Figure 19.

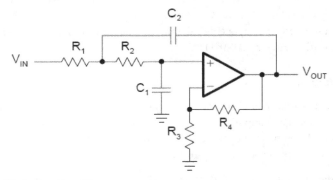

Figure 19. 2nd Order Low Pass Filter

For $R_1 = R_2$ and $C_1 = C_2$, the cut-off frequency of the circuit in Figure 19 is the same as that of Eq. 4. $R_3$ and $R_4$ are optional as they are required for separate gain settings as given in Eq. 5.

A 2nd order low pass filter is again recommended as compared to a 1st order one for the same reasons mentioned for a 2nd order high pass filter.

### 4.1.3. Band pass filtering for EMG

As mentioned previously, for the transmission of pure EMG, the high and low frequency noise should be deleted. For this purpose, only a specific band of frequency should be carried forward [20]. This can be made possible with the help of a band pass filter. A band pass filter response is shown in Figure 20.

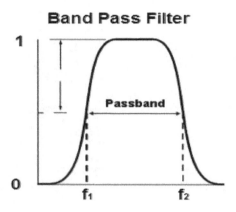

**Figure 20.** Band Pass Filter Response

The frequency region where the response of the EMG signal is '1' is called the 'passband' and in the case of band pass filter, it is between $f_1$ and $f_2$.

A band pass filter can be designed by connecting a low pass and a high pass filter in series. By selecting proper values of R and C, we can develop a band pass filter which can carry forward the most effective component of the EMG signal. It is recommended that for EMG, $f_1$ should be 65-70 Hz and $f_2$ be 150-180 Hz.

## 4.2. Amplification

After the signal has been filtered properly and a suitable band of EMG frequency is obtained, the next stage is amplification. The EMG signal obtained has to be powered up to a suitable level. The amplification of the EMG signal can be easily carried out with the help of a non-inverting amplifier, shown in Figure 21.

The gain of the amplifier is provided in the figure as 'Av'. The non-inverting amplifier is only used when the signal is being received from a single wire referenced to ground. Amplification can be done in stages in order to cater for chip requirements, by cascading them in series.

The EMG signal, as mentioned before, is very weak i.e. only 1-10 mV. For certain muscles, for which the signal response is very strong e.g. Biceps Brachii, a gain of 500-1000 can be enough. But for muscles, whose EMG response is weak e.g. Flexor Palmaris Longus (ring finger muscle), the gain settings should be very high i.e. 10000.

The proper gain setting solely depends upon the signal response observed from the subject's target muscle. It is to be noted that every subject gives a separate signal response. Some subjects will give weak responses as compared to others. So, in that case, appropriate gain value should be set once the subject's EMG signal response is properly observed.

## Non-Inverting Amplifier

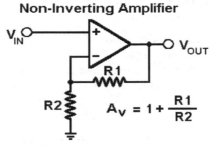

**Figure 21.** A Non-Inverting Amplifier

## 5. Control technique

In order to successfully achieve robotic prosthesis, an effective control technique is very important in order to drive the electric motors in the mechanism. With the advent of modern microcontroller technology, the control options available today have never been so effective.

For implementing the desired control to the motors, the amplified EMG signal in analog form has to be converted into digital format. After this, the motors are driven with the help of a microcontroller through the thresholding technique. These techniques will be discussed in detail in this section.

### 5.1. Analog to digital conversion

The digitization process of the analog signal is carried out with an Analog to Digital Converter (ADC). Nowadays, the ADC has become a common component of modern electronic devices. Their use has become highly varied and widespread. Before using the ADC, its specifications, advantages and limitations have to be analyzed in order to select the most appropriate one for the application. In the same way, important considerations have to be taken into account while converting EMG signals into digital format.

Control of the motor will be developed after the EMG signal is converted into digital format. A particular ADC has a specific range of conversion i.e. there are maximum and minimum levels defined for an ADC over which it can operate. An ADC can convert the analog signal over a certain number of bits. The number of bits which an ADC can convert is known as its "quantization scheme". If an ADC has a defined range and a quantization scheme of '*n-bits*', then the resolution of the ADC can be given as:-

$$V_{resolution} = V_{range}/(2)^n \qquad (6)$$

While converting an EMG signal into digital format, three specifications should be taken into account. 1) Quantization, 2) Range of conversion and 3) Sampling rate [21].

The number of bits, which an analog signal can be converted into digital format by an ADC, is known as quantization. The maximum amount of voltage an ADC can convert into digital quantized bits defines the range of an ADC. The sampling rate means the number of samples an ADC can convert in one second.

After the EMG signal has been amplified up to a suitable level, the range of an ADC should be selected so that it can comprehend a particular voltage level. The number of quantization bits is important, as they determine the resolution of the ADC. The more the number of quantization bits, the less will be resolution of the ADC; the more it will help in control purposes. The ADC sampling rate is also a key consideration. It should be kept as large as possible so that the data loss of EMG is kept at a minimum [21].

ADCs are now available as a peripheral with microcontroller chips and can give sampling rates greater than 1000 kSPS and quantization schemes of more than 24 bits.

## 5.2. Thresholding and motor drive

The control of robotic prosthesis is provided through the thresholding technique [21]. Once the signal is received in digital format, taking all necessary considerations as described before, a suitable threshold is applied to that particular quantized digital signal.

Before applying the threshold, the digital quantized signal is to be observed properly. A threshold value should then set be accordingly. It is recommended to set the threshold value to a point which is less than half the digital quantized output of the EMG signal. When the digital signal exceeds this threshold, the microcontroller should set an output pin to '1' and '0' otherwise [21]. E.g. if the maximum value of the digital quantized signal is 750 (decimal value) then we can set a threshold of 275. This signal is forwarded to an H-bridge or a motor driver in order to drive the respective electric motors of a robotic mechanism.

The motor driver should be designed or selected according to our requirements of electric motor. Usually a motor driver which can drive a 12V motor and handle up to 4A current can adequately meet requirements for a robotic arm.

## 6. Results and conclusions

A useful way of acquiring EMG signals and motor drive has been explained in this chapter. Modern microelectronics and controllers have enabled us to develop efficient control of prosthetic robotic mechanisms. To summarize the discussions made earlier, Figure 22 shows a block diagram depicting all the necessary steps required to achieve successful prosthesis.

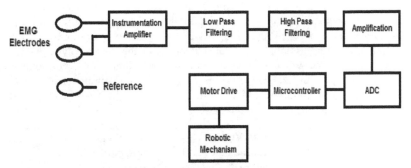

**Figure 22.** Block diagram indicating all steps for driving a robotic mechanism

As an example, we discuss the control of a robotic hand. There are two primary motions of the human hand, flexing and extending. For flexion, electrode should be placed on Flexor Digitorum Profundus and for extension; the electrode should be placed on Extensor Digitorum Communis [21]. As both muscles exhibit different signal patterns, therefore, a multi-channel input scheme should be employed, so that both signals are gathered independently. Both signals should be observed carefully and a suitable threshold should be set after filtering and amplification. The same procedure is to be followed in order to develop control of all the fingers of the robotic hand i.e. by placing EMG electrodes on specific muscles which control them, allowing us to classify different motions of the hand [22].

The signal observed from a subject with a moderate built is shown in Table 1. The amplification set for the detected EMG signals from the subject was 10,000. Table 1 provides the EMG signal response from each of the subject's fingers after amplification and threshold set for their control [21].

Size is a very important factor while designing an electronics circuit. A circuit occupying minimum space will be most appropriate in application. A size effective circuit will be easy to place and handle in a robotic mechanism. Advances in biomedical instrumentation have brought fruitful gains to robotic prosthetic technology. The ADS1298 is a 64 pin IC with 8 differential inputs with programmable gain amplifiers (PGAs) and a 24 bit ADC. The PGAs can provide a maximum gain of 12 but the 24 bit ADC quantization scheme is enough to process the EMG signal [23]. With all necessary peripherals attached to a single IC, the size of the whole circuitry can be reduced up to 95%.

Latest robotic researches have enabled us to design and create multi-degree of freedom robotic mechanisms [24]. A good mechanical design and apparatus is essential for efficient robotic prosthesis. Newer electronic components and materials have made robotic prosthesis more functional and adaptable. When we talk about materials, the perfect one should be lighter, durable, adjustable and comfortable for the user. Nowadays, carbon fiber frames are being employed as a solution to this matter. An example of a carbon fiber limb is the state of the art Ottoblock C-Leg. The C-Leg has a built in computer which analyzes data from various sensors and actuates the knee using a hydraulic cylinder.

When a human uses a robot, he desires to use his natural limb movements to control the mechanism. In order to achieve this, EMG provides the perfect assistance to allow a subject to make normal movements using a robotic apparatus, hence, efficient controllers and improved algorithms are essential for enhanced control of the device. Given the fact that EMG was introduced more than 30 years ago, the research community has a come a long way in coming up with innovative techniques, hardware solutions and advanced procedures to design, control and utilize these signals to produce resourceful prosthetic means to tackle disabilities and amputations effectively.

| S. No. | Finger/ Hand | Peak Voltage Reading before Contracting (V) | Peak Voltage Reading after Contracting (V) | Threshold Set (V) |
|--------|--------------|---------------------------------------------|--------------------------------------------|-------------------|
| 1 | Thumb (flexing) | 0.8 | 3.7 | 1.4 |
| 2 | Index (flexing) | 0.6 | 1.4 | 0.8 |
| 3 | Ring (flexing) | 0.2 | 2.5 | 0.7 |
| 4 | Pinkie (flexing) | 0.2 | 1 | 0.5 |
| 5 | Hand (flexing) | 0.2 | 5 | 1 |
| 6 | Hand (extending) | 0.15 | 4.5 | 0.8 |

**Table 1.** EMG signals observed and the threshold in terms of voltage [17]

## 7. Future challenges and directions

Scientists working on upper limb prosthesis define their goal in this field as to develop a 'simultaneous, independent, and proportional control of multiple degrees of freedom with acceptable performance and near "normal" control complexity and response time' [25]. The major challenges faced in prosthetics are: electromechanical implementation, use of EMG control signals and the interface between robotic and clinical communities [26]. Designing a robotic mechanism which is fully capable of integrating with human neuromuscular system is a tough proposition. The requirements can only be fulfilled if the apparatus is of light and flexible material with small but powerful actuators, size effective electronic components, sensors which can easily adapt with the skin and a long lasting battery life. Only then the machine will qualify to be used in everyday practical life [26].

The human hand has 20 degrees of freedom, and the body works in a unique variety of ways to tackle various hindrances placed in front of it. It is therefore, a great challenge to extract all of these motions from the body and utilize them in a resourceful way. Nowadays, two degree of freedom mechanisms are most common. To achieve further DOFs, sensors will be required to be placed at more sophisticated locations, which is a tough task.

The most important challenge of robotic prosthesis in rehabilitation is the feasibility of the mechanism. The apparatus should be comfortable, silent and aesthetically viable for the subject [26]. Our target should be the effective use of the robotic artificial limb on the physically disabled, not to waste our efforts in fruitless objects. Hence, for the reliability of the mechanism's implementation on the amputated population, clinician's approval should be made a part of the procedure.

Due to its practicality and noninvasiveness, SEMG proves to play a significant role in medical applications and rehabilitation prosthesis. However, the human machine interface will decide if the robotic mechanism will be used in everyday life application or not. It is very important to improve the Quality of Life (QOL) of elder and disabled population. It is believed that in the near future, "we will be able to replace entire limbs with prosthetics that can replicate one's own biological functions precisely, casting natural outward appearance and requiring minimum upkeep" [26].

Robotic researchers and biomedical engineers have been trying to combine their techniques to make the perfect biomechatronic mechanism. However, in order to ensure that challenges are met and to create a more smart and intelligent machine, communication between clinicians, users and engineers should be established on a greater scale.

## Author details

Muhammad Zahak Jamal

*National University of Sciences and Technology, Pakistan*

## Acknowledgement

The study was carried out at College of Electrical and Mechanical Engineering (CEME), NUST in collaboration with Armed Forces Institute of Rehabilitation Medicine (AFIRM). The author is highly indebted to Brig. Dr. Javaid Iqbal and Dr. Umer Shahbaz Khan for their help in the study and CEME for providing necessary funds to make this research possible. Special thanks to all colleagues and people who have willingly helped out with their abilities.

## 8. References

[1]  Alan G. Outten, Stephen J. Roberts and Maria J. Stokes (1996) "Analysis of human muscle activity", Artificial Intelligence Methods for Biomedical Data Processing, IEE Colloquium, London

[2]  Musslih LA. Harba and Goh Eng Chee (2002) "Muscle Mechanomyographic and Electromyographic Signals Compared with Reference to Action Potential Average Propagation Velocity", Engineering in Medicine and Biology Society, 19th Annual International Conference of the IEEE, Vol.3

[3]  Nissan Kunju, Neelesh Kumar, Dinesh Pankaj, Aseem Dhawan, Amod Kumar (2009) "EMG Signal Analysis for Identifying Walking Patterns of Normal Healthy Individuals" Indian Journal of Biomechanics: Special Issue

[4]  Carlo J. De Luca (1997) "Use of Surface Electromyography in Biomechanics" Journal of Applied Biomechanics, Vol.3

[5]  Carlo J. De Luca (2006) "Electromyography: Encyclopedia of Medical Devices and Instrumentation" (John G. Webster Ed.), John Wiley Publisher

[6]  Jarret Smith (2010) image title: "motor-unit-lg"

[7]   S.L. Pullman, D.S. Goodin, A.I. Marquinez, S. Tabbal and M. Rubin (2000) "Clinical Utility of Surface EMG" Report of the Therapeutics and Technology Assessment, Subcommittee of the American Academy of Neurology, Neurologly Vol. 55:171–177

[8]   Paul E. Barkhaus and Sanjeev D. Nandedkar (2000) "Electronic Atlas of Electromyographic Waveforms" Vol. 2, 2nd Edition

[9]   Nuria Masso, Ferran Rey, Dani Romero, Gabriel Gual, Lluis Costa and Ana German (2010) "Surface Electromyography and Applications in Sport" Apunts Medicina De L'Esport, Vol. 45: 127-136

[10] Dr. Scott Day "Important Factors in Surface EMG Measurement", Bortec Biomedical Incorporated

[11] (2008) "Bagnoli EMG Systems Users Guide", Delsys Incorporated

[12] Netter FH (1997) "Atlas of Human Anatomy" East Hanover, New Jersey: Novartis.

[13] Elaine Marieb and Katja Hoehn (2007) "Human Anatomy and Physiology" 7th Edition, Pearson Education

[14] Björn Gerdle, Stefan Karlsson, Scott Day and Mats Djupsjöbacka (1999) "Acquisition, Processing and Analysis of the Surface Electromyogram". In: U. Windhorst, H. Johansson, editors. "Modern Techniques in Neuroscience Research", Springer

[15] Carlo J. De Luca (2002) "Surface Electromyography: Detection and Recording", Delsys Incorporated

[16] D.J. Hewson, J.Y. Hoqrel and J. Duchene (2003) "Evolution in impedance at the electrode-skin interface of two types of surface EMG electrodes during long-term recordings" Journal of Electromyography and Kinesiology, Vol. 13, Issue 3 , pp. 273-279

[17] (2009) "Instrumentation Amplifier Application Note", Intersil Incorporated

[18] Gianluca De Luca (2001) "Fundamental Concepts in EMG Signal Acquisition", Delsys Incorporated

[19] P.R.S. Sanches, A.F. Müller, L. Carro, A.A. Susin, P. Nohama (2007) "Analog Reconfigurable Technologies for EMG Signal Processing" Journal of Biomedical Engineering, Vol. 23, pp. 153-157

[20] M. E. Van Valkenburg (1982) "Analog Filter Design", Holt, Rinehart & Winston

[21] Zahak Jamal, Asim Waris, Shaheryar Nazir, Shahryar Khan, Javaid Iqbal, Adnan Masood and Umar Shahbaz (2011) "Motor Drive using Electromyography for Flexion and Extension of Finger and Hand Muscles" 4th International Conference on Biomedical Engineering and Informatics, Vol. 3 pp. 1287-1291

[22] Sebastian Maier and Patrick van der Smagt (2008) "Surface EMG suffices to classify motion of each finger independently" Proceedings of MOVIC 2008, 9th International Conference on Motion and Vibration Control

[23] Datasheet ADS1298 "Low-Power, 8-Channel, 24-Bit Analog Front-End for Biopotential Measurements" Texas Instruments Incorporated.

[24] A. H. Arieta, R. Katoh, H. Yokoi and Y. Wenwai (2006) "Development of a Multi D.O.F Electromyography Prosthetic System Using Adaptive Joint Mechanism", Applied Bionics and Biomechanics, Vol. 3, Woodheads Publishing

[25] D. Edeer and C.W. Martin (2011) "Upper Limb Prostheses – A Review of the Literature with a Focus on Myoelectric Hands", WorksafeBC Evidence-Based Practice Group

[26] Brian Dellon and Yoki Matsuoka (2007) "Prosthetics, Exoskeletons, and Rehabilitation-Now and the Future" IEEE Robotics & Automation Magazine, March, 2007

# Virtual and Augmented Reality: A New Approach to Aid Users of Myoelectric Prostheses

Alcimar Barbosa Soares, Edgard Afonso Lamounier Júnior, Adriano de Oliveira Andrade and Alexandre Cardoso

Additional information is available at the end of the chapter

## 1. Introduction

During the past decades, great effort has been devoted to devise new strategies for the control of artificial limbs fitted to patients with congenital defects or who have lost their limbs in accidents or surgery [1-6]. Most of that work was dedicated to minimize the great mental effort needed to control the prosthetic limb, especially during the first stages of training. When working with myoelectric prosthesis, that effort increases dramatically. These devices use EMG signals (the electrical manifestation of the neuromuscular activation associated with a contracting muscle) collected from remnant muscles to generate control inputs for the artificial limb. As these devices use a biological signal to control their movements, it is expected that they should be much easier to control. However, the prosthesis control is very unnatural and requires a great mental effort, especially during the first months after fitting [2, 7, 8]. As a result, a number of patients give up the use of those devices very soon. To overcome those problems, different techniques have been tried as an attempt to devise better strategies for myoelectric control.

This chapter describes the advent of Virtual Reality (VR) systems to create training environments dedicated to users of prosthetic devices. Those VR systems generally simulate a prosthesis that can react to commands issued by the users. A sophisticated system proposed by the authors is also described. Known as *"The Virtual Myoelectric Prosthesis"*, the system is based on the use of EMG to control a virtual prosthesis in an Augmented Reality (AR) environment, in real time, providing the user with a more natural and intuitive training environment. The overall aim is to reproduce the operation of a real prosthesis, in an immersive AR environment, using a virtual device that operates in similar fashion to the real one. Also, the research team believes that, since real upper limb prostheses are relatively heavy and can become uncomfortable and cumbersome, especially during the first stages of fitting, the use of a virtually weightless and fully controllable device can help reducing the great physical and metal effort usually necessary, especially in the first trials.

## 2. Myoelectric prostheses

The human body has been considered a perfect machine, in which all parts work in harmony one with each other. Most of us can control this "machine" without much effort, until some disturbance caused by disease or injury results in loss of some of its functionality.

The absence of limbs caused by trauma or congenital disorders, can affect our lives profoundly. Simple tasks such as walking or dressing can become extremely difficult or even impossible to execute. There is no doubt that the best solution for the loss of a limb might be the development of some kind of genetic manipulation that stimulates the regeneration of tissue. However, while this is not possible, the best we can do is to restore some of the lost functionality by means of artificial limbs.

For centuries, mankind seek ways to replace lost limbs by mechanical devices. Several ancient designs can be found in museums and libraries. However, the first artifact to be formally named artificial limb was a Roman prosthesis, made of wood and bronze, which appeared around 300 BC [9]. During the Middle Ages, while the poor wore "wooden legs", which were simple, inexpensive and stable, the rich nobles used devices made of iron, which were more decorative than functional. In 1818 Peter Ballif designed the first prosthesis actuated by movements of healthy parts of the body. Before this, the upper limb prostheses were heavy and depended on an able hand for operation [10]. Thereafter, a number of experiments have been carried out seeking the "perfect prosthesis", a device that could be similar to what Wolfe had visualized in 1952 in his book *"New York: Random House"* [11]:

> *"They had perfected an artificial limb superior in many ways to the real thing, integrated into the nerves and muscles of the stump, powered by a built-in atomic energy plant, equipped with sensory as well as motor functions"*

As we know, to date, this prediction has yet to be completely materialized, but much has been done since then. Due to the great number of casualties of World War II, the government of the United States created in 1945 a program of research and development from which scientists and engineers were deeply involved in projects aimed at the development of artificial limbs for amputees [10].

Another fact that lead to the acceleration of the researches in the area, was the large number of congenital defects caused by the use of a drug called Thalidomide. As describe by Soares [10], it was synthesized by the German laboratory Chemie Grünenthal in 1957 and marketed worldwide between 1958 and 1962. This drug was prescribed to minimize sickness during pregnancy. The Thalidomide consumers were not warned that the drug could exceed the placenta affecting the fetus. This oversight had a catastrophic effect: drug abuse, especially during the first trimester of pregnancy, has killed thousands of babies. Those who survived experienced birth defects such as deafness, blindness, disfigurement, and especially the shortening or absence of members. Responding to this tragedy, several research centers intensified the efforts towards the design of artificial limbs as an attempt to improve the lives of those children.

Also, during that period, russian scientists had introduced a prosthetic hand controlled by a signal generated by the activity of remaining muscles from amputated limbs [8]. That type of control has been described as "myoelectric control" and the prosthesis, by extension, has been described as "myoelectric prosthesis".

## 2.1. Controlling strategies

The control of prostheses can be considered one of the most interesting challenges related to prosthetics. Ideally, a prosthetic limb should be controlled without any effort from the user, similar to the subconscious control of a natural limb.

Currently, there are two main strategies for controlling artificial limbs: biomechanical and bioelectrical. In the first, the motion of parts of the body results in the activation of the limb, whereas, in the latter, biosignals, generated from the electrical activity of muscles, are detected and interpreted in order to generate commands for controlling the prosthesis. Nevertheless, there is ongoing research seeking other forms of control based on more natural strategies, such as those that employ brain or neuronal activity together with sensory feedback [5-7, 12-14].

As described earlier, the first prostheses were generally passive devices that relied on intact parts of the body for their positioning and controlling. This extremely successful design allowed the user to control the device so that the movement of a part of the body was reflected in movements of parts of the prosthesis. Despite some modifications, this design remains basically the same nowadays, being the most popular control mechanism among users [10]. The reasons for such success are not well established, but according to Doeringer and Hogan [15] some of the key factors are: it results in a relatively inexpensive prosthesis; the final prosthesis is not too heavy; after training, the user begins to use the prosthesis as a natural extension of his body, having, for example, the notion of weight and size of the prosthetic limb. Kruit and Cool [16] described the main drawbacks: the mechanism of harnesses used to propagate the movements of the body is usually uncomfortable; the movement of the prosthesis requires significantly large forces; the number of control inputs is limited and thus the number of degrees of freedom of the prosthesis is also limited.

An alternative to the Body-Powered control is to employ the myoelectric control, which uses the electrical activity of muscle contraction (electromyographic signal) as a primary source of control. The prostheses that use this type of control typically do not require cables and, in some situations, there is no need for suspension straps. The operation of a myoelectric device can be summarized as follows: the brain sends commands, i.e., neuronal impulses that travel through nerves and reach the endplate of a given muscle, which, in turn, causes muscle contraction; The electrical muscle activity is then captured by electrodes (normally in a socket attached to the stump), interpreted by customized programs in a microcontroller, and used to activate the actuator of the prosthesis.

Many myoelectric prostheses employed a type of control called "two-site two-states", from which a pair of electrodes is placed on two distinct muscles. The contraction of one of these muscles produces the opening of the hand. The antagonist muscle is used in the same way to control the closing of the hand. As pointed out by Scott and Parker [8], this approach works in a manner analogous to the human body, i.e., two antagonistic muscles (or group of muscles) control the movement of a joint. However, as patients must learn to generate independent contractions of the muscles, which requires a high degree of concentration, the training can be lengthy and demand a lot of mental effort. There are also some situations in which it is not possible to find two available groups of muscles, or there might be more than one joint to be controlled. For these situations other controlling approaches have been developed [17]. For instance, the "one-site three-states", from which a little contraction of a muscle produces the closing of the hand, a strong contraction open it, and the lack muscle activity stops the hand. Figure 1 shows an example of a hand prosthesis controlled by electromyographic signals captured by four pairs of dome electrodes, distributed around the residual limb ([18]).

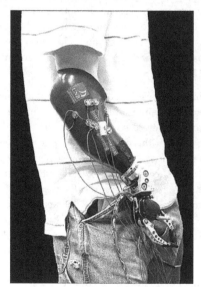

**Figure 1.** An experimental setup for a myoelectric prosthesis, developed at the University of New Bruswick, Canada (extracted from [18]).

Currently there are a number of methods using proportional control based on the electrical activity of muscles to control the speed, torque and position of prosthetic joints. However, due to the nature of the myoelectric signal, errors and inaccuracies may occur [19]. Myoelectric signals can be detected using basically two types of electrodes: surface electrodes positioned on the skin surface, and needle electrodes inserted in relevant positions of the muscle. In both cases the electrodes produce a difference of potential relative to a reference (typically another electrode located elsewhere on the body). This voltage is the result of an asynchronous activation of hundreds of muscle fibers. The signal is similar to a random noise whose amplitude is modulated by a voluntary input. Its shape depends on variables such as strength and speed of activation, positioning and types of electrodes used in its detection, electronic circuits used for acquisition, amplification and processing [20]. These factors make the translation of myoelectric activity into commands for a prosthetic limb a challenge. Moreover, the generation of myoelectric patterns must be learned by the user, and this is a task which requires concentration, regular training and a great amount of physical effort.

A common way of training an individual to generate myoelectric patterns is by using feedback software, which provides the user with visual feedback about the relation between the forces associated to the contraction with the amplitude of the generated myoelectric signal. The main drawback of this strategy is that it does not give the user feedback information or sense of proprioception. Recent studies have suggested that virtual and augmented reality [21] may be a relevant tool to address the limitations of conventional training techniques. The main advantage of this technique is that it can simulate the physical presence of the artificial limb in the real world, as well as in imaginary worlds. Moreover, some simulations may include additional sensory information, such as sound through speakers or headphones. It is also possible to include tactile information, generally known as force feedback, for the individual.

## 3. Virtual and augmented reality

Virtual Reality (VR) can be defined as an advanced computer interface where the user can, in real time, navigate within a tridimensional environment interacting with its virtual objects. Such interaction is achieved in a very intuitive and natural way. To do so, multisensory devices are supplied [22].

In order to illustrate this concept, consider Figure 2, in which a user is shown standing inside a research laboratory. However, since she is equipped with multisensory devices (Head Mounted Display – HMD and hand (glove) sensors), a computer-based system provides her the feeling of being steeped into a different environment.

The system, known as BioSimMER© (from Sandia National Laboratories) [23], is used to train rescue personnel to respond to terrorist attacks. The screen on the top shows the working environment displayed only for the eyes of the health professional and the virtual patient exhibits realistic symptoms. Such facilities are not supported by traditional computer interfaces.

Therefore, to achieve the high level of natural interface required by VR systems, it is important to provide the user with the feeling of immersion and the ability for interaction. To reach such requirements, VR developers must guarantee: 1) Real life 3D object images from the user's perspective; 2) The aptitude to track the user's motions, particularly his head and eye movements, and correspondingly adjust the images on the output device to reflect the change in perspective.

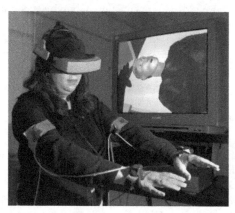

**Figure 2.** Experiment with virtual reality techniques and devices (extracted from [23]).

Augmented Reality (AR) is a technique that allows the integration of virtual objects within a real physical environment. Interaction is again supported by multisensory equipment. Essentially, a real scene, captured by a digital camera, is "augmented" with the insertion of virtual objects [24]. Figure 3 illustrates this concept.

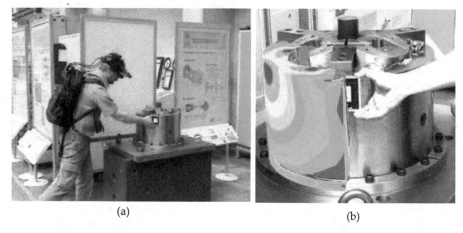

(a)                                                          (b)

**Figure 3.** An example of Augmented Reality extracted from [25]: (a) Positioning a fiduciary marker in mechanical part; (b) Heating distribution visualization through user's glasses.

In Figure 3(a), an engineer uses a fiduciary square marker to identify the heating distribution throughout a mechanical part, as shown in Figure 3(b). However, this "virtual" information can only be seen by him, through the equipment and glasses he carries.

A very well-known framework to support AR is the ARToolKit ([26]). It provides Computer Vision techniques to calculate position and orientation of a digital camera in relation to fiduciary markers. The augmentation is produced after a series of transformations, as shown in Figure 4. First, the real video image is transformed into a binary one. Then, this image is processed in order to determine square black regions (fiduciary markers – regions whose outline contour can be fitted by four line segments) containing an image pattern that is compared to patterns stored in a database. Next, the algorithm uses size-known squares and the pattern orientation as the base for the coordinates frame and to calculate the real position of the digital camera in relation to the physical marker. After that, the 3D objects are placed over the fiduciary markers, and the final image is sent to the display.

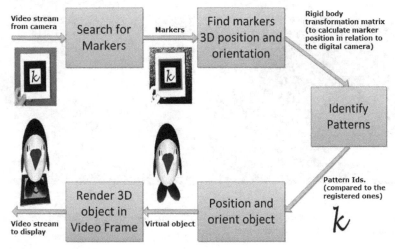

**Figure 4.** ARToolKit workflow.

Nowadays, VR and AR systems have been intensively used for training and simulation. According to [27] and [28], the main reasons for that are:

- It provides "Learning by doing" - according to pedagogical studies, the learning curve and the amount of knowledge acquired are intensified when the apprentice plays an active role during the process;
- It supports virtual and interactive experiments/simulations - replacing physical counterparts that could pose health hazard or even be too expensive in real life;
- It allows training to be executed outside classes and clinics; and
- It inspires creativity.

The strategies adopted by systems like the ARToolKit are promising and relatively simple to be incorporated into final applications. However, the need for physical markers can limit their application in many areas. Hence, an interface that is able to represent the real environment, capture movements and sounds and transforming them into actions to interact with virtual objects, have been the focus of many recent researches seeking a human-computer dialogue closer to natural. That's why the expression "natural user interface" has emerged as new computer interaction technology. It focuses on human abilities such as touch, vision, voice and higher cognitive functions, such as expression, perception and recall [29]. The main objective here is to give a physical meaning for the digital information. In so doing, data manipulation with the use of bare hands, gestures, voice commands and pattern recognition are supported.

Recently, Santos et al. [30] presented an application that uses gestures to interact with virtual objects in an Augmented Reality, based on Kinect© (a motion sensing input device developed by Microsoft Inc.). The application is not limited by environment, lighting or skin color and doesn't require fiduciary markers. The system allows the user to perform operations on menus and interact with virtual objects solely by hand gestures (Figure 5).

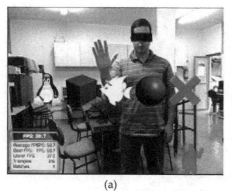 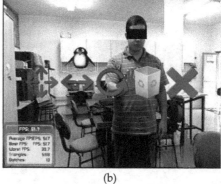

(a)                                                                               (b)

**Figure 5.** Natural User Interface with Augmented Reality: (a) User selecting menu options; and (b) User manipulating a virtual object (extracted from [30]).

In recent past years, it has been observed a steady growth in the use of Virtual and Augmented Reality in health care [31, 32]. There a number of examples in the literature. However, to ilustrate the technique, let's take two examples into account.

Payandeh and Shi [33] presented a mechanics-based interactive multi-modal environment designed to teach basic suturing and knotting techniques for simple skin or soft tissue wound closure. Two haptic devices are used for force-feedback, simulating the experience of suturing a real tissue (Figure 6).

That realist feeling was provided by a number computer-based techniques, such as mass-spring system, to simulate the deformable tissue (skin), mechanics-based techniques to simulate the deformations of a linear object (the suturing material) and collision detection for the interactions between the soft tissue and the needle. Figure 7 shows a pre-wound scene (a) and the result after the virtual suture (b).

Virtual and Augmented Reality have also been studied as a tool for phobia treatment [34]. As an example, consider the system describe in [35]. The project, which is accompanied by a psychologist, aims to design a system to gradually confrontate the patient with his object phobia. Clinical studies have shown that some patients cannot handle, or even do not evolve in the treatment, if exposed to a real arachnid in the initial sessions. Thus, AR is used to present the patient with virtual objects that reminds a spider (like a cartoon) and this object, gradually, becomes a very 'realistic' virtual one (with photorealism modeling techniques). Figure 8(a) shows a potential user wearing the system apparatus and Figure 8(b) shows the image seen by the user.

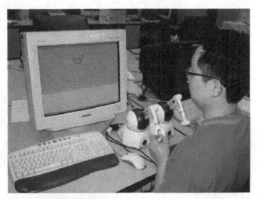

**Figure 6.** VR multi-modal experimental setup for simulating surgical sutures (extracted from [33]).

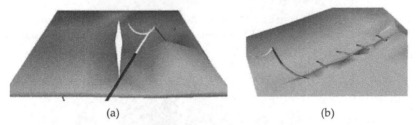

(a)                                                         (b)

**Figure 7.** (a) Virtual pre-wound tissue for suturing; (b) Virtual wound closed (extracted from [33]).

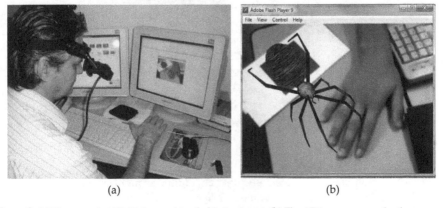

(a)                                                         (b)

**Figure 8.** (a) User wearing HMD for arachnophobia treatment; (b) The AR image, as seen by the user.

Based on the discussions above, we can infer that VR and AR incorporate a number of features with great potential to overcome some of the difficulties associated with the training of prosthetic users.

## 4. Virtual prostheses

As described earlier, great effort has been devoted to devise new strategies for the control of artificial limbs fitted to patients with congenital defects or who have lost their limbs in accidents or surgery. In general, the devices do not properly resemble the real counterpart, do not react in the same manner, do not provide proper feedback and cannot be controlled using the "natural" interfaces, i.e., signals emanated from the central nervous system. Therefore, a number of difficulties arise when a new user tries to control an artificial limb, since he/she will have to devise a completely new strategy to generate input signals for the prostheses, so that it will act according to his/her wishes. This leads to a lengthy, tiring, and sometimes frustrating, training period. That is true for the great majority of the strategies for prosthesis control that have been designed to date.

Recently, a number of research groups turned their attention to VR and AR, in an attempt to overcome some of those problems. Although many works can be found in the literature, we have chosen just a few to illustrate the concept.

Pons *et al.* [36] describe the use of VR to support the training process for a multifunctional myoelectric hand prosthesis (MANUS) capable of generating up to four grasping modes (cylindrical, precision, lateral and hook grasps, in addition to wrist pronation-supination).

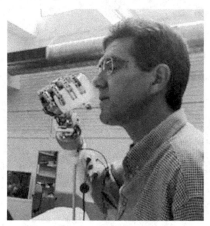

**Figure 9.** One of the MANUS users performing a combined cylindrical grasp and wrist rotation (extracted from [36]).

As expected, multifunctional prostheses pose an additional problem for users: the more dexterous the device, the higher the number of command channels required to control it. As a result, a large number of different EMG commands, generally obtained by extra EMG channels, are required for successful management of the prosthesis. To minimize the number of channels, the authors proposed a three-bit ternary EMG command strategy. The users were asked to produce EMG bursts (by sudden contraction of a single muscle) and, if proper EMG thresholds could be defined, each burst was classified in three different levels. Each of those three levels were then given the digital values "0", "1" or "2" (no signal, low, high), corresponding to one ternary bit. In so doing, if the user generates three bits, he/she could generate up to 27 different combinations (commands) from a single muscle. However, since the commands starting with "0" (i.e., "0XY") were not valid, the three-bit ternary strategy allowed the generation of 18 effective commands. This means that, from a single muscle, the user could control up to 18 different functions/actions of the prosthesis. However, that is no easy task to learn. Hence, a special training device, based on VR simulation of the multifunctional prosthesis, was created to enable the learning of that "EMG command language". Only after the training process was finished, the prosthesis was fitted and real manipulative operation started. The authors report that all of the volunteers were able to successfully perform basic commands after about 45 minutes.

In similar fashion, Resnik *et al.* [37] show the use of VR as an aiding tool for training users of advanced upper-limb prostheses. The device known as DEKA Arm (DEKA Research & Development Corporation) allows users 10 powered degrees of movement (Figure 10a). A VR environment program (Figure 10b) was created to allow users to practice controlling an avatar, using the controls designed to operate the DEKA Arm in the real world.

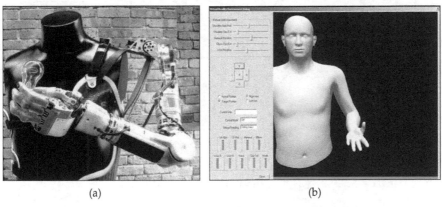

(a)                                                                      (b)

**Figure 10.** (a) DEKA Arm displayed on manikin; (b) VR avatar (extracted from [37]).

The authors report that the VR environment allows a gradual acclimatization to the arm, as the experience with the arm-control scheme prior to use of the physical arm allows a staged introduction of the new elements of the system. However, the system did not allow for interaction with virtual objects, i.e., it was not possible, for instance, the manipulation of an object with the virtual hand. Nevertheless, the system proved to be an important asset for upper-limb users who must master a large number of controls and for those who need a structured learning environment, due to cognitive deficits.

## 4.1. The virtual myoelectric prosthesis

Although VR has been extensively used as an aiding tool for users of prosthetic devices, the interaction with the virtual world still needs to be improved, in order to provide a real immersive training environment. To do so, the research group headed by the authors, have developed new techniques for VR interaction and for detection and processing of EMG signals, in order to extract the correct commands issued by the user which, in turn, could be used to control the movements of a device in a VR environment [21, 28, 30, 38]. However, although a purely non-immersive VR environment showed some good results, it was thought that an Augmented Reality (AR) environment would provide a more realistic experience. Hence, an AR environment was designed so that images of the virtual device (the prosthesis) are combined with images of the real world, providing a realistic environment for training upper limb prosthetic users [39]. A simplified block diagram of the system is shown in Figure 11.

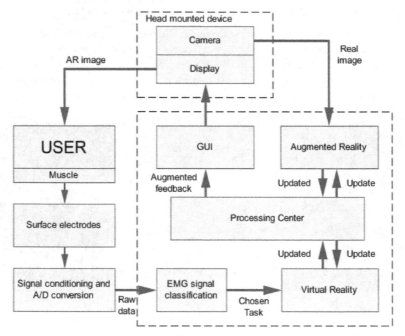

**Figure 11.** The authors' approach for a Virtual Myoelectric Prosthesis (extracted from [39]).

In the system, the user is fitted with a head mounted device that includes a camera, for capturing the real images of the user's view point, and a display to show the mixed images (augmented: real and virtual). The EMG signals are collected and processed to generate inputs to the VR unit [21]. A processing center decides when to update both the virtual arm (Figure 12) and the augmented reality image, to further send them to the graphics user interface (the head mounted display).

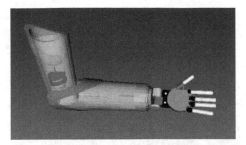

**Figure 12.** A Virtual Prosthesis designed by the authors.

During operation, the camera captures the image and locates a marker at the user's shoulder. The algorithm then searches for a virtual object that corresponds to such marker (Figure 13) and inserts it into the real world, captured by a camera.

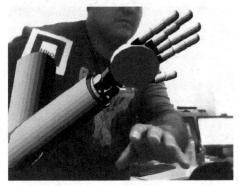

**Figure 13.** Image of a virtual object combined with the real world scene – an outsider point of view (extracted from [39]).

As described in [39], the control inputs for the AR environment are generated by EMG signals, collected from remnant muscles. The raw EMG signal, detected by surface electrodes is conditioned and processed to find out which movement the user wants to perform. To do so, the areas of activity in the EMG data were detected (windowing) and the resulting signal was then processed to generate a set of features used by an artificial neural network classifier. Basically, each EMG contraction was represented by a set of Auto-Regressive (AR) coefficients calculated according to a modified algorithm described in [38]. According to the authors, the choice of a neural network as a classifier was due to its ability to learn and later recognize signals as being part of the same class of movement in real time. Also, depending on the level of amputation, different users may generate different levels of contractions of the remaining part of the limb, for the same class movement. Besides, even if a single user performs only isometric or isotonic contractions, there will not be two identical contractions for the same movement. The neural network was trained with four classes of movements (elbow flexion, elbow extension, wrist pronation and wrist supination). The results showed a near perfect performance of the classifier (95% to 100% rate of success). The output of the neural network is then used as control input (position and motion) to the virtual device, which can be rendered and mixed with the real world scene, as shown in Figure 14.

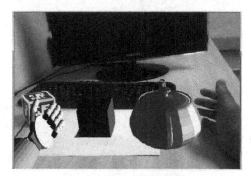

**Figure 14.** User's point of view within the AR environment (extracted from [39]).

Note that this system allows the user to interact within the virtual environment - the virtual myoelectric prosthesis can touch and grab other virtual objects embedded in the real scene (such as the cube and the kettle in Figure 14). Also, a strong cognitive feedback is provided by this real time mixture of virtual objects with the real environment, given the feeling that it is almost possible to touch the virtual arm with the real one, and vice-versa.

## 5. Conclusion

This chapter presented an overview on the search of human beings for artificial devices capable of restoring, if not all, at least part of the functionality lost when we are affected by diseases, congenital disorders or trauma that results in the loss of a limb. Focusing on upper limb prosthesis, a series of sophisticated technical solutions have been proposed during the past decade to design devices whose behavior and control approach that of their healthy natural counterparts. However, as described along this chapter, operating a highly complex artificial limb is not a simple task. This is especially true for myoelectric multifunctional prostheses with many degrees of freedom. Since the necessary control commands, in most instances, can be very different from the "natural" commands, learning how to produce them is extremely difficult and time consuming. With the advent of Virtual and Augmented Reality, those technologies have been proposed as relevant tools to address some of the limitations of conventional training techniques. It is possible to design a virtual device very similar, in shape and behavior, to a real one. Also, it is even possible to collect commands from the real world (EMG signals generated by remnant muscles) and use them as inputs to control the actions of a virtual prosthesis in an Augment Reality Environment, according to the training stage of the user, or any other setup defined by the therapist. In so doing, those techniques allow for a considerable reduction of physical and metal efforts usually necessary to master the control of a prosthetic device.

## 6. Future directions

Despite the progress achieved so far, the authors believe that, as technology advances, the use of virtual and augmented reality for controlling myoelectric prostheses should also undergo continuous improvements. These future developments should be focused on issues such as: (i) improving the modeling of the virtual devices, in order to increase the sense of realism when compared to actual prostheses; (ii) new adaptive protocols for controlling the virtual prosthesis, so that it could emulated different strategies and different joint actuators; and (iii) the design of new devices to provide physiological feedback, allowing the user to "feel" what the virtual prosthesis is actually doing, thus, increasing the feeling of a complete mix between the real and virtual worlds.

## Author details

Alcimar Barbosa Soares* and Adriano de Oliveira Andrade
*Laboratory of Biomedical Engineering, Faculty of Electrical Engineering,*
*Federal University of Uberlândia, Brazil*

Edgard Afonso Lamounier Júnior and Alexandre Cardoso
*Laboratory of Computer Graphics and Virtual Reality, Faculty of Electrical Engineering,*
*Federal University of Uberlândia, Brazil*

## Acknowledgement

The authors would like to express their gratitude to "Coordenação de Aperfeiçoamento de Pessoal de Nível Superior" (CAPES - Brazil), "Conselho Nacional de Desenvolvimento Científico e Tecnológico" (CNPq – Brazil) and "Fundação de Amparo à Pesquisa do Estado de Minas Gerais" (FAPEMIG – MG – Brazil) for the financial support.

## 7. References

[1] Davoodi R, Loeb GE. Real-Time Animation Software for Customized Training to Use Motor Prosthetic Systems. IEEE Transactions on Neural Systems and Rehabilitation Engineering 2012; 20(2) 134-142.

[2] Scheme E, Englehart K. Electromyogram Pattern Recognition for Control of Powered Upper-Limb Prostheses: State of the Art and Challenges for Clinical Use. Journal of Rehabilitation Research & Development 2011; 48(6) 643–660.

[3] Simon AM, Hargrove LJ, Lock BA, Kuiken TA. Target Achievement Control Test: Evaluating Real-time Myoelectric Pattern-recognition Control of Multifunctional Upper-limb Prostheses. Journal of Rehabilitation Research & Development 2011; 48(6) 619–628.

* Corresponding Author

[4]   Su Y, Fisher MH, Wolczowski A, Bell GD, Burn DJ, Gao RX. Towards an EMG-Controlled Prosthetic Hand Using a 3-D Electromagnetic Positioning System. IEEE Transactions on Instrumentation and Measurement 2007; 56(1) 178-186.

[5]   GEAKE TH. An Advanced Feedback System for Myoelectrically Controlled Prostheses. MPhil Thesis. School of Computer Science and Electronic Systems, Kingston University, UK, 1994.

[6]   Patterson PE, Katz JA. Design and Evaluation of a Sensory Feedback System that Provides Grasping Pressure in a Myoletric Hand. Journal of Rehabilitation Research and Development 1992; 29(1), 1-8.

[7]   Paciga JE, Richard PD, Scott RN. Error rate in five-state myoelectric control systems. Medical and Biological Engineering and Computing 1980; 18(3) 287-90.

[8]   Scott RN, Parker PA. Myoeletric Prosthesis: State of the Art. Journal of Medical Engineering & Technology 1988; 12 143-151.

[9]   Lamb DH, Law H. Upper-Limb Deficiencies in Children – Prosthetic, Orthotic and Surgical Management. Boston, USA: Little, Brown and Company, 1987.

[10]  Soares AB. Shape Memory Alloy Actuators for Upper Limb Prostheses. PhD Thesis. University of Edinburgh; 1997.

[11]  Childress DS. Powered Limb Prostheses: Their Clinical Significance. IEEE transactions on biomedical engineering 1973; BME-20(May) 200-207.

[12]  Cram JR. The history of surface electromyography. Applied Psychophysiology and Biofeedback 2003; 28 81-91.

[13]  Horowitz S. Biofeedback Applications: A Survey of Clinical Research. Alternative and Complementary Therapies 2006; 12(6) 275-281.

[14]  Oskoei MA, Hu H. Support vector machine-based classification scheme for myoelectric control applied to upper limb. IEEE Transactions on Biomedical Engineering 2008; 55(Aug) 1956-1965.

[15]  Doringer JA, Hogan N. Performance of Above Elbow Body-Powered Prostheses in Visually Guided Unconstrained Motion Tasks. IEEE Transactions on Biomedical Engineering 1995; 42(6) 621-631.

[16]  Kruit J, Cool JC. Body-powered Hand Prosthesis with Low Operating Power for Children. Journal of Medical Engineering & Technology 1989; 13 129-133.

[17]  Andrade AO. Methodology for EMG Signal Classification for the Control of Artificial Members. MSc Dissertation. Federal University of Uberlândia, Brazil; 2000.

[18]  Kyberd PJ, Lemaire ED, Scheme E, MacPhail C, Goudreau L, Bush G, Brookeshaw M. Two-degree-of-freedom Powered Prosthetic Wrist. Journal of Rehabilitation Research & Development 2011; 48(6) 609–618.

[19]  Hoff LA. Errors in Frequency Parameters of EMG Power Spectra. IEEE transactions on biomedical engineering 1991; 38 1077-1088.

[20]  O'Neill PA, Morin EL, Scott RN. Myoletric Signal Characteristics from Muscles in Residual Upper Limbs. IEEE Transactions on Rehabilitation Engineering 1994; 2 266-270.

[21] Soares AB, Andrade AO, Lamounier Jr EA, Carrijo R. The Development of a Virtual Myoelectric Prosthesis Controlled by an EMG Pattern Recognition System Based on Neural Networks. Journal of Intelligent Information Systems 2003; 21(2):127-41.

[22] Cardoso A, Kirner C, Lamounier Jr EA, Kelner J. Technologies to the development of virtual and augmented reality systems; Editora Universitária da UFPE, Portuguese version, 2007.

[23] Sandia National Laboratories. BioSimMER - Virtual Life-saver. http://www.sandia.gov/media/NewsRel/NR1999/biosim.htm (accessed 25 April 2012).

[24] Kirner C, Kirner TG. Virtual Reality and Augmented Reality Applied to Simulation Visualization. In: El Sheikh, A.A.R.; Al Ajeeli, A.; Abu-Taieh, E.M.O. (Org.). Simulation and Modelling: Current Technologies and Applications. 1st ed. Hershey-NY: IGI Publishing, 2007; 1 391-419.

[25] Weidlich D, Scherer S, Wabner M. Analyses Using VR/AR Visualization. IEEE Computer Graphics and Visualization 2008; Sept/Oct 84-86.

[26] GNU General Public License. http://www.gnu.org/licenses/gpl.html (accessed 5 February 2007).

[27] Azuma R, Bailot Y, Behringer R, Feiner S, Julier S, MacIntyre B. Recent Advances in Augmented Reality. IEEE Computer Graphics and Applications 2001. 21(6) 34-47.

[28] Soares AB, Lamounier Jr EA, Lopes K, Andrade AO. Augmented Reality: A Tool for Myoelectric Prostheses. In: ISEK 2008: XVIIth Congress of the International Society of Electrophysiology and Kinesiology, ISEK2008, 18-21 June 2008, Niagara Falls, Canada.

[29] Liu W. Natural User Interface - Next Mainstream Product User Interface. In: 2010 IEEE 11th International Conference on Computer-Aided Industrial Design & Conceptual Design (CAIDCD), 17-19 November 2010; 1 203 - 205.

[30] Santos E, Lamounier Jr EA, Cardoso A. Augmented Reality Interaction with Kinect Device. In: Proceedings of the XIII Brazilian Symposium on Virtual and Augmented Reality, SVR2011, 23-26 May 2011.

[31] Riva G. Virtual Reality for Health Care: The Status of Research. CyberPsychology & Behavior 2002; 5(3) 219-225.

[32] Marescaux J, Rubino F, Arenas M, Mutter D, Soler L. Augmented-Reality–Assisted Laparoscopic Adrenalectomy. The Journal of the American Medical Association 2004; 292(18) 2214-2215.

[33] Payandeh S, Shi. F. Interactive Multi-Modal Suturing. Virtual Reality 2010; 14(4) 241–253.

[34] Juan MC, Alcaniz M, Monserrat C, Botella C, Banos R, Guerrero B. Using Augmented Reality to Threat Phobias. IEEE Computer Graphics and Aplications 2005; 25(6) 31-37.

[35] Lima L, Cardoso A, Nakamoto P, Lopes E, Lamounier Jr EA. Development of a Computer Tool to Aid Arachnophobia Treatment with Augmented Reality. In: Proceedings of the XIII Brazilian Symposium on Virtual and Augmented Reality, SVR2011, 23-26 May 2011.

[36] Pons JL, Ceres R, Rocon E, Levin S, Markovitz I, Saro B, Reynaerts D, Van Moorleghem W, Bueno L. Virtual reality training and EMG control of the MANUS hand prosthesis. Robotica 2005; 23 311-317. doi:10.1017/S026357470400133X

[37] Resnik L, Etter K, Klinger SL, Kambe C. Using Virtual Reality Environment to Facilitate Training with Advanced Upper-Limb Prosthesis. Journal of Rehabilitation Research & Development 2011; 48(6) 707–718.

[38] Soares AB, Veiga ACP, Andrade AO, Pereira AC, Barbar JS. Functional Languages in Signal Processing Applied to Prosthetic Limb Control. Systems Analysis Modelling Simulation 2002; 42 1377-1389.

[39] Lamounier Jr EA, Lopes K, Cardoso A, Soares AB. Using Augmented Reality Techniques to Simulate Myoelectric Upper Limb Prostheses. Journal of Bioengineering & Biomedical Science 2012; S1:010. doi:10.4172/2155-9538.S1-010

# Permissions

The contributors of this book come from diverse backgrounds, making this book a truly international effort. This book will bring forth new frontiers with its revolutionizing research information and detailed analysis of the nascent developments around the world.

We would like to thank Dr. Ganesh R. Naik, for lending his expertise to make the book truly unique. He has played a crucial role in the development of this book. Without his invaluable contribution this book wouldn't have been possible. He has made vital efforts to compile up to date information on the varied aspects of this subject to make this book a valuable addition to the collection of many professionals and students.

This book was conceptualized with the vision of imparting up-to-date information and advanced data in this field. To ensure the same, a matchless editorial board was set up. Every individual on the board went through rigorous rounds of assessment to prove their worth. After which they invested a large part of their time researching and compiling the most relevant data for our readers. Conferences and sessions were held from time to time between the editorial board and the contributing authors to present the data in the most comprehensible form. The editorial team has worked tirelessly to provide valuable and valid information to help people across the globe.

Every chapter published in this book has been scrutinized by our experts. Their significance has been extensively debated. The topics covered herein carry significant findings which will fuel the growth of the discipline. They may even be implemented as practical applications or may be referred to as a beginning point for another development. Chapters in this book were first published by InTech; hereby published with permission under the Creative Commons Attribution License or equivalent.

The editorial board has been involved in producing this book since its inception. They have spent rigorous hours researching and exploring the diverse topics which have resulted in the successful publishing of this book. They have passed on their knowledge of decades through this book. To expedite this challenging task, the publisher supported the team at every step. A small team of assistant editors was also appointed to further simplify the editing procedure and attain best results for the readers.

Our editorial team has been hand-picked from every corner of the world. Their multi-ethnicity adds dynamic inputs to the discussions which result in innovative outcomes. These outcomes are then further discussed with the researchers and contributors who give their valuable feedback and opinion regarding the same. The feedback is then collaborated with the researches and they are edited in a comprehensive manner to aid the understanding of the subject.

Apart from the editorial board, the designing team has also invested a significant amount of their time in understanding the subject and creating the most relevant covers. They scrutinized every image to scout for the most suitable representation of the subject and create an appropriate cover for the book.

The publishing team has been involved in this book since its early stages. They were actively engaged in every process, be it collecting the data, connecting with the contributors or procuring relevant information. The team has been an ardent support to the editorial, designing and production team. Their endless efforts to recruit the best for this project, has resulted in the accomplishment of this book. They are a veteran in the field of academics and their pool of knowledge is as vast as their experience in printing. Their expertise and guidance has proved useful at every step. Their uncompromising quality standards have made this book an exceptional effort. Their encouragement from time to time has been an inspiration for everyone.

The publisher and the editorial board hope that this book will prove to be a valuable piece of knowledge for researchers, students, practitioners and scholars across the globe.

# List of Contributors

**Javier Rodriguez-Falces, Javier Navallas and Armando Malanda**
Department of Electrical and Electronic Engineering, Public University of Navarra, Pamplona, Spain

**Penka A. Atanassova and Nedka T. Chalakova**
Department of Neurology; Medical University, Plovdiv, Bulgaria

**Borislav D. Dimitrov**
Department of General Practice, Division of Population Health Sciences, Royal College of Surgeons in Ireland, Dublin, Republic of Ireland
Academic Unit of Primary Care and Population Sciences, University of Southampton, Southampton, United Kingdom

**Begoña Gavilanes-Miranda**
Faculty of Physical Activity and Sport Science, University of Basque Country, Vitoria, Spain

**Juan J. Goiriena De Gandarias**
Faculty of Medicine, University of Basque Country, Bilbao, Spain

**Gonzalo A. Garcia**
Biorobotics Department, TECNALIA, Bilbao, Spain

**Runer Augusto Marson**
Laboratory of Biomechanics and Kinesiology, Sport Center, Federal University of Ouro Preto, Minas Gerais, Brazil
Laboratory of Biomechanics, Research Institute of Physic Capacity of the Army, Rio de Janeiro, Brazil

**Leandro Ricardo Altimari, José Luiz Dantas, Marcelo Bigliassi and Thiago Ferreira Dias Kanthack**
Group of Study and Research in Neuromuscular System and Exercise, CEFE - State University of Londrina, Brazil

**Antonio Carlos de Moraes**
GPNeurom - Laboratory of Electromyography Studies, FEF - State University of Campinas, Brazil

**Taufik Abrão**
Department of Electrical Engineering, CTU - State University of Londrina, Brazil

**Takeshi Tsujimura**
Department of Mechanical Engineering, Saga University, Japan

**Sho Yamamoto**
Department of Mechanical Engineering, Saga University, Japan

**Kiyotaka Izumi**
Department of Mechanical Engineering, Saga University, Japan

**R.K. Jain, S. Datta and S. Majumder**
Design of Mechanical System Group/Micro Robotics Laboratory, CSIR-Central Mechanical Engineering Research Institute (CMERI), Durgapur, West Bengal, India

**César Ferreira Amorim**
University of City of São Paulo-UNICID, São Paulo - SP, Brazil

**Runer Augusto Marson**
Sports Center, Federal University of Ouro Preto, Ouro Preto - MG, Brazil

**Gabriela Winkler Favieiro and Alexandre Balbinot**
Federal University of Rio Grande do Sul (UFRGS), Graduate Program in Electrical Engineering (PPGEE), Department of Electrical Engineering, Instrumentation Laboratory, Porto Alegre, Rio Grande do Sul, Brazil

**Muhammad Zahak Jamal**
National University of Sciences and Technology, Pakistan

**Alcimar Barbosa Soares and Adriano de Oliveira Andrade**
Laboratory of Biomedical Engineering, Faculty of Electrical Engineering, Federal University of Uberlândia, Brazil

**Edgard Afonso Lamounier Júnior and Alexandre Cardoso**
Laboratory of Computer Graphics and Virtual Reality, Faculty of Electrical Engineering, Federal University of Uberlândia, Brazil

Printed in the USA
CPSIA information can be obtained
at www.ICGtesting.com
JSHW011445221024
72173JS00004B/944

9 781632 411617